A CLINICAL MANUAL OF ORTHOPEDIC TRACTION TECHNIQUES

GERHARD SCHMEISSER, Jr., M.D.

Chief of Orthopedic Surgery,
Baltimore City Hospitals.
Assistant Professor of Orthopedic Surgery,
Johns Hopkins University School of Medicine.

ILLUSTRATED BY ROBERT KERN

W. B. SAUNDERS COMPANY

PHILADELPHIA – LONDON – 1963

PREFACE

DESPITE so many dramatic achievements, recent advances in surgical technology have failed to cope with problems posed by the increasing number of patients whose brain, chest or abdominal injuries preclude early surgical management of their coincidental major fractures. The degree of comminution and displacement of many fractures created by modern machinery frequently defies the best surgical skill available. Even in the cleanest hospitals, postoperative osteomyelitis continues all too commonly to devastate the maimed. Orthopedic traction, if properly utilized, is a safe and rewarding alternative in the treatment of many major fractures. Its potential has not been exploited because its success depends upon a high level of understanding and cooperation, not only of the responsible surgeon and his assistants but also of the orderlies, aides, technicians, student nurses, practical and registered nurses, house officers, and medical students, who care for the patient while the responsible surgeon is elsewhere.

Thus the purpose of this monograph is to facilitate the better use of traction for major injuries by presenting the pertinent principles, preferred equipment, manner of assembly and maintenance in such a fashion as to be intelligible and useful to all members of the hospital team. It is designed as a working manual and not as a comprehensive textbook. For more extensive study of the subject, the reader is referred to Dr. Carlo Scuderi's *Atlas of Orthopedic Traction Procedures* (St. Louis, C. V. Mosby Company), the standard fracture text-

books, and the specific references mentioned in relevant sec-
tions. Traction techniques for injuries of the hand and
forefoot are omitted, since their value is more limited and
they do not represent a hospital team problem in patient care.
Traction techniques for contractures of various joints and for
congenital dislocation of the hip are also beyond the scope of
this book. Such techniques may be improvised easily by one
who grasps principles.

The author will be particularly pleased if this manual
finds its way into nurses' stations and treatment rooms and
into the hands of students and house officers. Size, binding
and format were selected in an effort to meet the practical
needs of this group. Semidiagrammatic line drawings are
used in the interest of both clarity and economy.

In an abbreviated and mimeographed form this manual
has proved helpful in the instruction of many classes of medical students and nurses at the Johns Hopkins and Baltimore
City Hospitals. It has also proved of value to the attending
surgeon, both as a reference manual when ordering a traction
assembly by telephone and as a guide when personally fitting
together an unfamiliar arrangement.

G. S.

ACKNOWLEDGMENTS

THE AUTHOR is grateful to the late Dr. James P. Miller, at once the most delightful and provocative of teachers, for the inspiration to produce this monograph. The support and encouragement of Drs. Robert A. Robinson and Mark M. Ravitch are greatly appreciated. Particular thanks are rendered to Mrs. Corine Carr for her patient typing and copying. Without the artistic skill of Mr. Robert Kern and the wisdom and cooperation of the W. B. Saunders Company, this book would not exist.

CONTENTS

OBJECTIVES AND LIMITATIONS

Although traction may occasionally be used to distract or to immobilize a diseased joint, its usual purposes are to align the fragments of broken bones and to maintain alignment until union occurs. With any fracture, the same goals may be obtained by various combinations of the techniques of manual closed reduction, plaster cast immobilization, open surgical reduction, internal metallic fixation, and traction. Experienced judgment is required in making the best selection of these alternatives for any particular phase of the treatment. In a fracture for which traction could be used, its advantages are the avoidance of surgically induced bone devascularization, the avoidance of infection, and the greater potential for joint and muscle exercise than is afforded by plaster encasement. The prime disadvantage is prolonged recumbency, usually in a hospital. This difficulty does in fact preclude the use of traction techniques in certain types of patients. On the other hand, it should be appreciated that recumbency is not adequate justification to enforce or even to tolerate physical idleness.

EXERCISE

In order to offset some of the disadvantages of prolonged recumbency and to take advantage of the amount of exercise permitted by the traction arrangement, attending personnel should instruct and supervise the patient in an organized exercise program. On the day following their injuries, most patients should be encouraged to feed and wash themselves. They should be given ample encouragement but only limited physical assistance in these activities. If the apparatus is properly adjusted, the patient, if properly instructed in the use of the trapeze, will usually be able to lift himself to facilitate change of linen or use of the bedpan without disturbing alignment. For at least a few minutes several times a day, he should put every joint, except the ones immediately above and below the fracture, through a full range of motion. Deep breathing and abdominal setting exercises should be practiced from the start. Muscle-setting exercises over the injured segment of the extremity should be practiced as soon as pain and swelling permit. Limited and careful range of motion exercises of the joints immediately above and below the fractures may usually be initiated after callus appears on the x-ray. Certain modifications of the traction apparatus, as illustrated in succeeding chapters, facilitate these exercises. Crutch walking without weight bearing on the injured leg is frequently delayed in post-traction patients because of muscular weakness in the sound leg and in the upper extremities. This delay can be prevented while the patient is still recumbent by a program of lifting 5- to 10-pound weights with the arms and lifting a similarly weighted sandal with the uninjured leg. Supervision of the traction patient's physical activity can be performed only by the personnel in constant contact with him. For this reason it is mandatory that the house staff, nurses, aides and orderlies understand the exercise program as well as possible.

Reference

DeLorme, T. L., and Watkins, A. L.: Progressive Resistance Exercise: Technic and Medical Application. New York, Appleton-Century-Crofts, Inc., 1951.

PRINCIPLES OF TRACTION AND COUNTERTRACTION

Although a detailed knowledge of the physics of therapeutic traction is unnecessary for clinical personnel, three important principles should be recognized.

1. The appendage must be supported and stretched in such a direction as to align the bone fragments within it. In practice, traction is exerted on the distal fragment, aligning it with the less manageable proximal fragment, rather than vice versa.

2. The extremity must not be overstretched, thereby causing excessive distraction of the bone fragments.

3. The stretching forces must remain constant in amount and direction with respect to each other until the broken bones knit.

The two stretching forces must be applied and maintained with minimal discomfort and damage to the patient. At the same time at least some movement of the patient in bed must be possible. With one exception (Fig. 2) all arrangements illustrated in this text employ one or more weights for the traction force. In most cases the patient's body weight, resting on an inclined surface and tending to slide down that surface, constitutes the countertraction force.

Bed boards should always be interposed between mattress and springs in order to eliminate sag. Furthermore, the mattress should be firm, thereby increasing the efficiency of the inclined surface.

Exceptions to the technique of obtaining countertraction by tilting the bed are that illustrated in Figure 2, in which the half-ring pressed against the ischial tuberosity supplies the countertraction, and several other arrangements whereby a pulley on the traction cord transfers the direction of pull to a vertical rather than an oblique line. When, as in most cases, the traction force is exerted in an oblique line, the tilt of the bed in the opposite direction must be relative in degree to the amount and direction of the traction force. Only in this fashion can the amount of stretch on the extremity be kept constant. A common error is inadequate tilt, causing inadequate countertraction, in which case the patient migrates toward the traction force. Ultimately the knot on the traction bow impinges against the framework at the foot of the bed. The final result is loss of effective stretch on the injured section of the extremity. This situation can be corrected only by sliding the patient away from the traction force and increasing the tilt of the bed with higher shock blocks. With a little effort the patient can usually be taught to maintain himself in the proper position even if the bed is somewhat inadequately tilted. Another common error is indiscriminate elevation of the back rest of the bed. When there is traction on a lower limb, undue elevation of the back rest will promote migration of the patient toward the foot of the bed, with the unhappy consequences already mentioned.

3

EQUIPMENT

All too frequently traction equipment becomes a nuisance to everyone concerned. Total cost is unncessarily high, storage seems to require a vast amount of space which readily becomes a disorganized maze of hardware, small but vital parts are lost, and the orderly invariably appears with the wrong item of equipment. The basic error in such circumstances is the purchase and use of complex traction devices, each of which is designed for only a single type of traction. As this book illustrates, one type of equipment can be made to serve almost all traction purposes well. The octagonal tubular aluminum overhead frames with their attachments are recommended. This equipment is highly versatile, manageable and reliable, and is now available from several manufacturers at relatively reasonable prices. It can be stored disassembled on a special cart or in almost any closet that can accommodate an 8-ft. pole. It requires no oiling or other maintenance and is practically indestructible. A special virtue of octagonal poles is that a clamped joint between two such poles will not slip under stress. Round poles have proved troublesome in this respect, a difficulty which might be overcome by more powerful clamps. Despite these recommendations, therapeutic principles are constant regardless of equipment. Round poles, ordinary pipe, and even 2 x 4-in. wood beams can be used with equal results but with decidedly more effort.

Pulleys should be of ball-bearing type and should have clamps which can be attached to a pole from the side rather than threaded over the end. Clamps on the ends of the 5½-ft. upright poles should swivel 360° whereas the clamps on the ends of the short poles used for crossbars should not swivel at all. Clamps with 16 facets rather than 8 are preferable because of the greater ease of attachment in different positions.

Experience has shown that braided nylon cord ⅛ in. thick makes the best traction cord. It is readily stored in a small space and is of adequate strength. Traction cord should be purchased in quantity since it should not be used more than once.

Except in special arrangements, hospital beds for traction patients should be ones in which at least the back and knee elevations can be operated by separate cranks at the foot of the bed. It should also be possible to elevate only the foot portion of the springs and mattress. Fracture beds with built-in Bradford frames to support the patient when the mattress is lowered for use of the bedpan are particularly useful for patients with unstable fractures of the pelvis or with upper extremity or other injuries that preclude use of a trapeze.

Shock blocks of approximately 6- and 10-in. heights are a very necessary part of these traction arrangements. Bed jacks are helpful in elevating beds onto these blocks but are seldom as available as strong men. The doctor who lifts the end of a bed while facing it and bending over rather than by backing up to it and lifting with the help of his hip and knee extensors is himself foolishly seeking a disability.

Bed boards are an important feature of any traction arrangement. The most serviceable bed boards are not large and cumbersome sheets of plywood or fiberboard but are simple slats of wood approximately ¾ in. thick, 10 in. wide and as long as the width of the mattress. These slats are arranged parallel and close together between mattress and springs. If properly oriented, they do not interfere with the cranking up of the knee rest or back rest. Furthermore, they are easily stored and transported.

Details of lower extremity traction splints are discussed on page 38. Other specific items of equipment are discussed in relevant chapters.

KNOTS

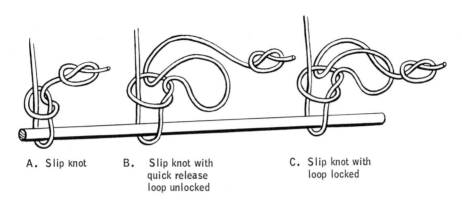

A. Slip knot   B. Slip knot with   C. Slip knot with
                    quick release   loop locked
                    loop unlocked

Fig. 1. Varieties of slip knots.

The simple slip knot or variations of it are very satisfactory under most traction circumstances. If a loop is drawn through the knot as illustrated, the knot may be released immediately by pulling on the free end. To prevent unintentional release the free end may be placed through the loose loop. In occasional situations the clove-hitch, which can be tied under tension, is quite useful (see Figure 33). Knots such as the granny, which are both insecure and difficult to untie, are particularly troublesome with traction arrangements.

To prevent unraveling, free ends should always be finished off with an overhand knot rather than wrapped with adhesive tape. The latter technique is time consuming initially and ultimately untidy. There is no advantage in the similarly messy practice of concealing the knot itself under a wad of tape.

ENCIRCLING DEVICES

Special Features

When an encircling device, such as a head halter, ankle hitch, or anklet, is used to obtain traction on a part of the body, the skin under that device is necessarily subjected to pressure. In general, such skin does not tolerate the constant pressure created by 10 or more pounds of traction for more than 24 hours. On the other hand, the skin tolerates the pressure exerted by much higher forces for a few hours, provided all pressure is removed after that time. Unstable fractures of the cervical spine or femur usually require fairly high and constant traction forces. Therefore, if it is elected initially to use an encircling device in the treatment of one of these injuries, one should switch within a few hours to some other technique of immobilization. Obviously, the change should be effected as gently as possible. For these reasons head halters and pelvic traction belts are used most widely not for fractures but for painful arthritis, degenerated or ruptured intervertebral discs, and sore ligaments and muscles. In such cases either light or intermittent traction is permissible.

Traction Splint and Anklet for Temporary Immobilization of a Fractured Femur

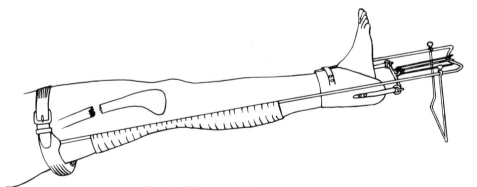

Fig. 2.   Traction splint and anklet.

Equipment

      1 reversible half-ring traction leg splint (Keller-Blake)
      1 heel rest
      1 hand towel with 8 spring clips (or large safety pins), or 2-ft. length of medium width stockinette
      1 traction anklet with 3-in. spreader bar or 1-yd. length of muslin
      2 yd. of traction cord

For many years, various modifications of the Thomas traction splint have proved efficacious and even life-saving in the initial immobilization of fractures of the shaft of the femur. By its proper use, further laceration of muscle by the raw bone ends with consequent additional internal hemorrhage and shock is minimized. In this apparatus the patient is easily transported, and x-rays can be obtained in the casualty receiving station with minimal disturbance. Ultimately, definitive care requires either surgical fixation or a more elaborate traction arrangement.

Purchase may be obtained on the lower leg by a skeletal pin, by skin traction, or by a traction anklet. An anklet is preferred in this situation, since it is quickly applied with minimal manipulation and is quite satisfactory for a few hours. If a commercial traction anklet is not readily available, a suitable substitute can be improvised quickly from a length of stockinette or muslin tied about the ankle as illustrated. Generous padding should be used.

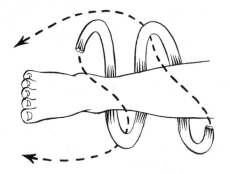

Fig. 3. Ankle traction hitch.

Traction splints of the Keller-Blake type with neoprene-padded half-rings and with hinges at the junctions of the half-ring with the side bars are ideal. They are reversible for use with either the right or left leg and are easy to apply. It is important that a tight hammock in the form of a stockinette sleeve or a hand towel with its edges pinned about the side bars be used to support the leg in the splint. The limb should be placed in the split with manual support under the knee and a firm, steady pull on the foot.

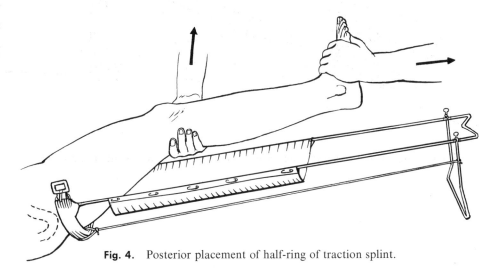

Fig. 4. Posterior placement of half-ring of traction splint.

The half-ring, oriented posteriorly, should lie in the gluteal fold engaged against the ischial tuberosity in such a fashion as to facilitate effective countertraction. Frequently, owing to the padding about the hinges, the half-ring does not stay in the proper depressed position. Under these circumstances the correct position may be maintained by tying a length of traction cord under tension from the center of the half-ring to some fixed point near the narrow end of the splint. Fixed traction is obtained by tying the muslin strips under tension around the end of the traction splint. Adequate pull can usually be achieved in this manner. Increased traction, if necessary, may then be obtained by twisting these cords with a tongue blade.

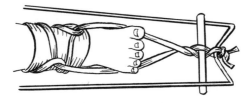

Fig. 5   Spanish windlass for increased traction.

The distal end of the splint must be supported at an adequate height to minimize anterior angulation of the bone fragments. When a commercial heel rest that attaches to the bottom of the traction splint is not available, a box of plaster serves the same purpose adequately.

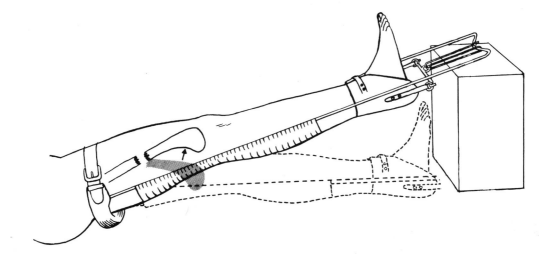

Fig. 6.   Alignment of femoral fragments by elevation of the distal end of the splint.

Pelvic Sling for Fractures of the Pelvis

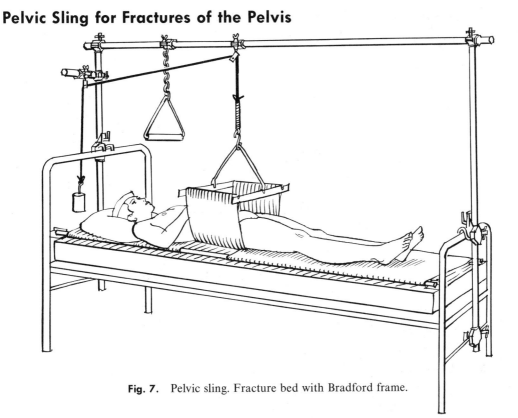

Fig. 7.   Pelvic sling. Fracture bed with Bradford frame.

Although this sling has enjoyed some popularity, its use is not recommended. Theoretically, it should be useful if the innominate bones are displaced laterally like the pages of an open book. In actual practice, if the sling is correctly arranged to compress the pelvis, great difficulty is encountered in using the bedpan. For this act, the sling is usually released or slid cephalad, thereby losing effective compression. Patients with fractures of the pelvis with slight displacement convalesce satisfactorily without a sling when they are placed on a fracture bed with a built-in Bradford frame, which permits the mattress to be lowered for the bedpan without disturbing the patient. When displacement is adequate to require reduction, closed reduction with a carefully applied spica cast after the manner of Watson-Jones suffices. Occasionally, open reduction and internal fixation are necessary. An alternative method, consisting of applying traction to hooks inserted through the iliac crests, has been reported by Almond and Vernon. If the displacement of one of the innominate bones is cephalad rather than lateral, a pelvic sling may actually be harmful. In this case, skeletal traction applied to the lower limb on the involved side may suffice (see Figure 31).

References

Almond, G., and Vernon, E.: Iliac skeletal cross traction. A method of treatment of "oyster-shell" pelvis. J. Bone & Joint Surg., *41B:*779, 1959.

Dommisse, G. F.: Diametric fractures of the pelvis. J. Bone & Joint Surg., *42B:*432, 1960.

Noland, L., and Conwell, H. E.: Acute fractures of pelvis. Treatment and results in 125 cases. J.A.M.A., *94:*174, 1930.

Watson-Jones, R.: Dislocations and fracture dislocations of the pelvis. Brit. J. Surg., *25:*773, 1938.

Pelvic Traction Belt for Relief of Low Back Pain in the Absence of Fracture or Dislocation

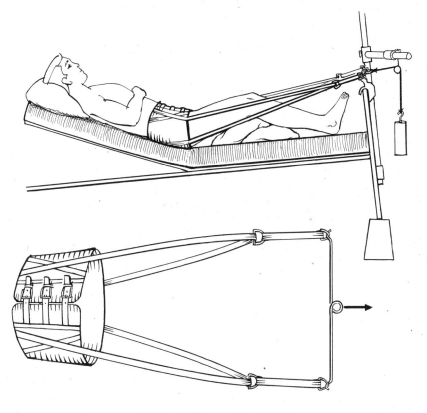

Fig. 8. Pelvic traction belt.

Equipment

- 1 pelvic traction belt with large spreader
- 1 yd. of traction cord
- 1 weight carrier and 20 pounds of weights
- 2 5½ ft. upright posts each with a swivel end clamp and an upper and lower toggle clamp
- 1 9 in. traction arm with end clamp
- 1 pulley with clamp assembly
- 1 8 ft. plain tube
- 1 trapeze with clamp and hook
- 2 large pillows
- 2 10-inch shock blocks

The pelvic traction belt or, when such belts are not available, bilateral Buck's extension, continues to be used for relief of low back pain simply because it frequently seems to help. It is naive to assume that sufficient tensile forces can be applied by these mechanisms to affect the vertebral articulations or paravertebral muscles directly. Instead, they probably work by discouraging the patient from climbing out of bed unnecessarily.

Careful positioning of the patient and adjustment of the bed are necessary to make the patient comfortable and to transmit as much traction force as possible to the vertebral articulations and paravertebral muscles. Bed boards beneath the mattress are essential. Shock blocks of adequate height under the foot of the bed are necessary to provide countertraction. The back rest should be elevated slightly but not so much as to slide the patient down in bed. Pillows should be placed beneath the knees to relax the hamstrings. The knee break should not be cranked up as a substitute for the use of pillows, since it tends to block transmission of traction force to the pelvis. Finally, a trapeze within the patient's reach helps him to shift about.

Head Halter for Relief of Neck Pain or for Temporary Immobilization of a Cervical Fracture or Dislocation

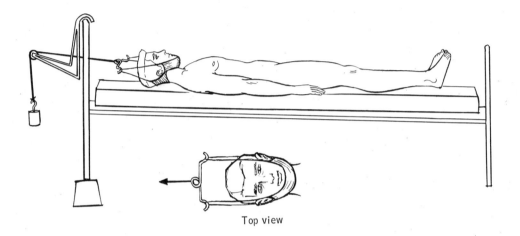

Top view

Fig. 9.   Head halter traction.

Equipment

> 1 head halter with 6-in. spreader bar
> 1 yd. of traction cord
> 1 weight carrier and 5 pounds of weights
> 1 adjustable Buck's extension hook
> 2 6-in. shock blocks

Head halter traction is used frequently for relief of neck pain or of cervicogenic shoulder and arm pain. The halter can be removed with impunity at any time, or the line of pull may be adjusted without risk in any direction that gives relief. At least some inclination of either the back rest or the entire bed must be used to prevent the patient from sliding toward the pulley. Cervical traction devices are currently available which consist of adjustable pulleys, with appropriate clamps, designed to attach the unit to the upper end of the back rest of the bed. With such a device the back rest may be cranked up or down without altering the traction forces. Simpler devices, such as adjustable Buck's extension hooks, which attach to the headboard of the bed, lack this flexibility. Part of an overhead traction frame arranged as in Figure 12 serves the same purpose just as well.

Halters, depending upon their design, secure purchase on the chin and occiput or, in some cases, the forehead and occiput. Seldom will the underlying skin tolerate more than 5 pounds of pull for prolonged periods. The author prefers the expendable models consisting of 2 reinforced padded gauze strips and 2 cord loops. One gauze strip is placed behind the occiput and the other under the chin. If a standard halter is not available, one can be hastily improvised from a piece of stockinette split longitudinally, as described by Froimson.

Head halter traction is also useful for temporary immobilization of necks with suspected fractures or dislocations until confirmatory x-rays have been taken. Thereafter, if the cervical spine is judged to be unstable, skeletal tong traction is preferred because of the larger traction forces that can be exerted. When head halter traction is used under this circumstance, the traction must not be released or the head lifted, turned or pushed without great care, lest neurologic injury occur. In this case, if the patient is riding up in bed and therefore must be moved downward, the attendants should lift the torso in this direction, allowing the head to trail behind. Turning the patient on his side is obviously exceedingly dangerous.

References

Crooks, F., and Birkett, A. N.: Fractures and dislocations of the cervical spine. Brit. J. Surg., *31*:252, 1944.
Forsyth, H. F., Alexander, E., Davis, C., and Underdal, R.: The advantages of early spine fusion in the treatment of fracture-dislocation of the cervical spine. J. Bone & Joint Surg., *41A*:17, 1959.
Froimson, A.: Stockinet head halter. J. Bone & Joint Surg., *43A*:1241, 1961.

SKIN TRACTION

Special Features

Skin traction achieved by attaching various types of adhesive strips over large areas of an extremity withstands about 10 pounds of pull for about 4 weeks before slipping. This form of traction is particularly suitable for younger children, because of their fast healing time and the light forces required for reduction and immobilization. Furthermore, it presents no hazard of bone infection or damage to the epiphyseal growth apparatus. On the other hand, most young patients and some older ones exhibit an unfortunate tendency to disarrange the elastic bandage and to tunnel with their fingers under the traction tape. Skin traction cannot be used easily to control rotation. It cannot withstand the magnitude and duration of forces frequently required, and it should not be used over injured skin.

Details of Application

Ordinary adhesive tape or moleskin, properly applied, serves adequately for Buck's extension or any other type of skin traction. However, many surgeons prefer the more recently available synthetic sponge strips backed with strong fabric. Some of these products are coated with adhesive gum, whereas others rely upon the friction of the sponge surface to secure purchase. It should be recognized that all of these devices irritate the skin to some extent; therefore, they should not be applied over an area where insertion of a skeletal traction pin or an incision might be necessary. Thus, if Buck's extension is applied for temporary immobilization of a fractured hip, the tape should not run above the knee. If surgery is not anticipated, the tape may run higher but should not extend quite as high as the level of the fracture. If it does extend to or above the level of the fracture, part of the pull on the tape will be transmitted via the soft tissues to the proximal fragment rather than just the distal fragment, thereby reducing efficiency. The strips of tape should not overlap both in back and in front of the extremity; instead a small strip of skin should be left uncovered to permit swelling and to prevent constriction should the traction tape tend to slip down the extremity. Within these limitations the traction tape should cover as much skin as possible in order to minimize the pull on each square unit of skin surface.

Shaving the extremity prior to application of the tape is usually not necessary to secure good adhesion, provided the skin is well cleaned with ether. On the other hand, if the limb is particularly hirsute, removal of the tape is likely to be particularly uncomfortable. For this reason the author prefers to shave such extremities, preferably with electric hair clippers, with care to avoid scratches or very close shaving which are likely to cause folliculitis under the tape. Tincture of benzoin, despite its traditional use in many institutions, actually does not improve the bond of most kinds of tape. Further-more, it does not really protect the skin. Therefore, unless specified by the manufac-turer of the specific type of tape, its use offers no advantage. The elastic bandage used to improve the bond of tape to skin must be wrapped snugly enough to do the job, but without wrinkles and not so tightly as to cause distal swelling. A few turns of the band-age about the foot inside the free ends of the traction tape also reduce this problem. The malleoli and particularly the tendo-achillis usually need some protective padding.

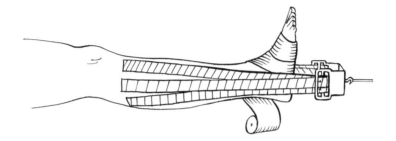

Fig. 10.   Skin traction with converging adhesive tape strips.

If strips of adhesive tape are used for traction, they must converge into double or triple thickness at the spreader in order to take the stress of 10 pounds for any pro-longed period.

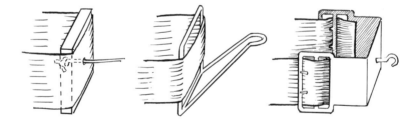

Fig. 11.   Spreader blocks. *A*, Perforated wood block; *B*, Wire; *C*, Baxter.

Several types of spreader blocks are available, each with minor advantages. The traction tape should be divided into separate medial or lateral strips only if a spreader with buckles is used. Selection of a spreader with width equal to that of the ankle is more important than design.

For Temporary Immobilization of a Fractured Hip or Immobilization Following Reduction of a Dislocated Hip

Buck's Extension

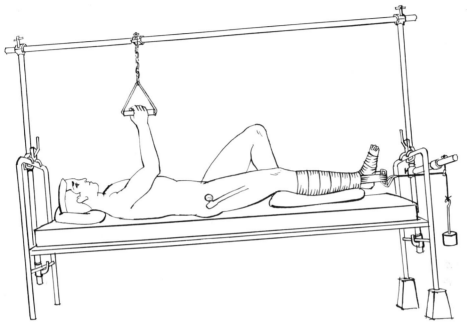

Fig. 12.   Buck's extension with overhead trapeze.

Equipment

    1 strip of commercial sponge traction tape or 2 wide strips of moleskin or 6 long strips of 2-in. adhesive tape
    1 4-in. elastic bandage
    1 spreader block
    1 yd. of traction cord
    1 weight carrier and 10 pounds of weights
    2 5½ ft. upright posts each with a swivel end clamp and an upper and lower toggle clamp
    1 18-in. traction arm with end clamp
    1 8-ft. plain tube
    1 trapeze with clamp and hook
    1 large pillow
    2 6-in. shock blocks

    Buck's extension to the lower limb is widely used for any condition of the knee, femur or hip joint in which partial immobilization with light traction force is desired. When greater traction force is necessary than is possible with skin traction, a pin through the calcaneus or distal tibia and fibula may be used as illustrated in Figure 28. An adjustable Buck's extension hook may be used to carry the traction cord over the end of the bed, but this device is cumbersome to store and offers no advantage over a pulley and crossbar attached to part of an overhead traction frame. Furthermore, the trapeze can then be attached to the same overhead frame rather than to a separate gibbet. The foot of the bed must be elevated by shock blocks to provide countertraction.

The patient can then move himself easily by pulling down on the trapeze with his hands while pushing down on the mattress with the foot of his uninjured leg. In moving the patient cephalad, assistance is provided by moving the patient's torso, allowing the leg in traction to drag behind. A pillow should be placed beneath the lower leg, but not under the heel. In the correct position the pillow prevents friction on the heel, provides flexion of the knee, and facilitates transmission of the traction force proximally. Elevation of the knee rest should not be permitted, since it tends to block transmission of this force above the knee. The degree to which partial turning of the patient may be permitted depends upon the stability of the fracture.

Russell's Traction

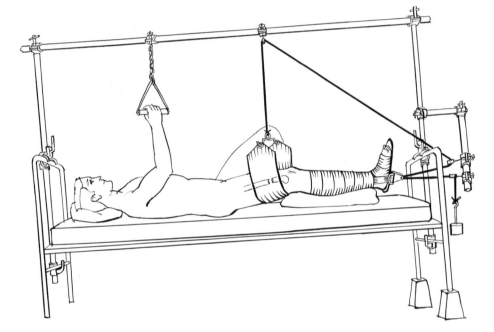

Fig. 13.   Russell's traction with overhead frame.

Equipment

 1 strip of commercial sponge traction tape or 2 wide strips of moleskin or 6 long strips of 2-in. adhesive tape
 1 4-in. elastic bandage
 1 foot plate with an attached pulley and two buckles
 1 stockinette covered felt sling 6 in. wide and 18 in. long with 6-in. spreader bar (Fig. 15)
 4 yd. of traction cord
 1 weight carrier and 10 pounds of weights
 2 5½ ft. upright posts each with a swivel end clamp and an upper and lower toggle clamp
 1 18-in. traction arm with end clamp
 1 9-in. traction arm with end clamp
 3 pulleys with clamp assemblies
 1 8 ft. plain tube
 1 trapeze with clamp and hook
 1 large pillow
 2 6-in. shock blocks

Russell's traction is simply a refinement of Buck's extension distinguished by the addition of a supporting sling behind the knee. One or more pillows are placed under the knee and lower leg, both to prevent the heel from pressing on the mattress and to maintain the correct degree of knee flexion. The arrangement may be used for the same conditions as Buck's extension but has greater usefulness for fractures of the femoral shaft in children and for tibial plateau fractures in adults. As with Buck's extension, when heavy traction force is desired it may be obtained by virtue of a skeletal pin through the calcaneus or distal tibia and fibula. Pull may be exerted on both the sling and the foot plate by a single cord and weight carrier as illustrated, or independent adjustments can be obtained by separate traction cords and weight carriers. This last arrangement is sometimes called "split Russell's" (Fig. 29).

Effective countertraction requires the use of shock blocks under the foot of the bed in order to incline it away from the traction force. The patient can then shift himself in bed by pulling on the trapeze and by pushing down on the mattress with his good foot. Assistance of the patient's movements is provided by lifting the patient rather than his leg. In this apparatus the patient must not turn from the waist down.

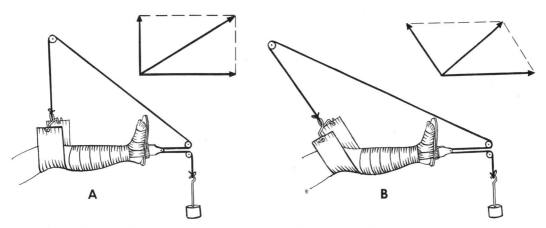

A   B

Fig. 14.   Size and direction of the resultant traction force in Russell's traction in relation to the position of the overhead pulley.

As shown by parallel-of-force diagrams, the direction of the resultant effective traction does not coincide with that of either the axis of the lower leg or the line of pull of the sling. The lower end of the bed cannot be cranked up without altering the direction of the traction. Furthermore, the size of the effective traction force is increased by moving the overhead pulley caudad and decreased by moving it cephalad. However, maintenance of the proper position of the sling requires a vertical or slightly cephalic orientation of this pulley. The correct position for the sling in relation to the leg depends upon the location and angulation of the fracture.

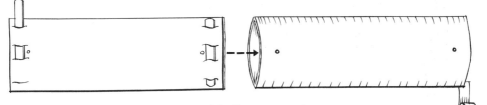

Fig. 15.   Felt sling construction.

The felt sling is fashioned from a ½-in. thick strip of saddler's felt 6 in. wide and 18 in. long. It is slit several times near each end and tongue blades are threaded through these slits to prevent curling of the sling when under tension. After the felt has been slipped into the tube stockinette and the ends have been closed with adhesive tape, holes are made to receive the spreader bar. Use of a sling without a spreader bar tends to constrict the leg unless the sling is considerably longer than the circumference of the leg.

References

Lee, W. E., and Veal, J. R.: The Russell extension method in the treatment of fractures of the femur. A review of the anatomical results obtained in a group of fifty-one cases. Surg. Gynec. & Obst., 56:492, 1933.
Lowry, T. M.: The physics of Russell traction. J. Bone & Joint Surg., 17:174, 1935.
Russell, R. H.: Fracture of the femur. A clinical study. Brit. J. Surg., 11:491, 1924.
Wendel, A.: Extracapsular fractures of the femur in the aged. A contribution to the merits of Russell treatment. J. Bone & Joint Surg., 13:616, 1931.

Bryant's Traction for Immobilization of a Fractured Femur in a Child 1–3 Years Old

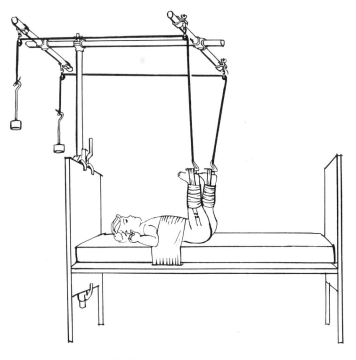

Fig. 16. Bryant's traction.

Equipment

    2 strips of commercial sponge traction tape or 4 wide strips of moleskin or 12 long strips of
      2-in. adhesive tape
    2 3 in. elastic bandages
    2 small spreader blocks
    4 yd. of traction cord
    2 weight carriers and 15 pounds of weights
    1 5½ ft. upright post with a swivel end clamp and an upper and lower toggle clamp
    1 36-in. traction arm
    2 traction bars with center clamps
    4 pulleys with clamp assemblies
    1 restraint of vest type

Although Bryant's traction is a very effective means of immobilizing and treating a
fractured femur in a young child, its use entails a definite risk of compromised circulation and resultant Volkmann's contracture of the foot and lower leg of either the
injured or the opposite limb. This risk is significantly greater in older children; therefore, Bryant's traction should not be used on children over about 3 years of age.
Children under 1 year of age with fractured femurs are preferably treated without any
form of traction. The feet of any child in Bryant's traction should be checked frequently
for pallor, loss of sensation, loss of toe motion, or other signs of circulatory embarrass-
ment, particularly during the first 48 hours. If such signs occur, the circumferential
dressings must be loosened, the traction force reduced and the legs brought down to an
angle at which circulation is restored. Frequently the circulation will be quite good with
the legs supported at a moderate angle created by cranking up the knee and foot portions of the bed (see Figure 17). This form of traction is very useful with children
slightly older than the ideal age for Bryant's traction.

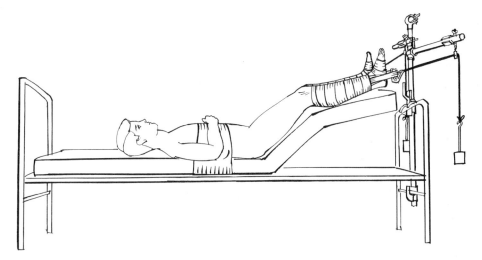

Fig. 17.   Bilateral high angle Buck's extension.

When Bryant's traction is used in an orthodox fashion, both legs are suspended
vertically with sufficient weight in the carriers that the buttocks barely lift off of the
mattress. A vest type restraint is sometimes desirable to anchor the active child to the
bed in such a fashion that he cannot twist around. The occasional practice of suspending only one leg does not restrain an active child adequately and tends to produce

angulation at the fracture site. With the apparatus arranged as in Figure 16, the child may be lifted a few inches off the bed in order to change the linen or clean his back without disturbing the actual traction force. The practice of merely tying the spreader block to an overhead frame without the use of weights and pulleys is not recommended, since it does not permit lifting the child without loss of traction force.

Whenever practical, location of the traction weights and other apparatus at the head end rather than the foot of the bed helps to clear passageways and to remove temptation from meddlers.

References

Cole, W. H.: Results of treatment of fractured femurs in children with especial reference to Bryant's overhead traction. Arch. Surg., *5:*702, 1922.
Nicholson, J. T., Foster, R. M., and Heath, R. D.: Bryant's traction: A provocative cause of circulatory complications. J.A.M.A., *157:*415, 1955.

Buck's Extension with Balanced Suspension for a Fractured Femur in a Child 4–8 Years Old

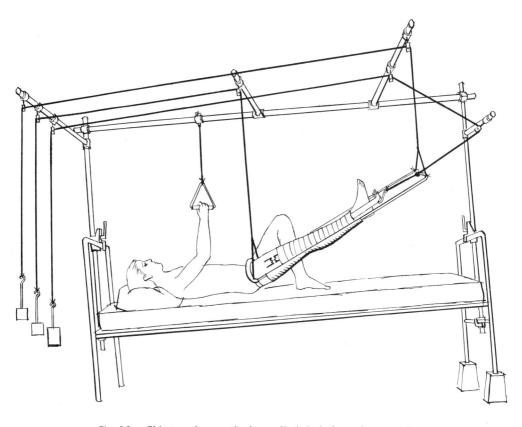

Fig. 18.   Skin traction on the lower limb in balanced suspension.

Equipment

    1 strip of commercial sponge traction tape or 2 wide strips of moleskin or 6 long strips of 2-in. adhesive tape

    2 3-in. elastic bandages

    1 spreader block

    1 small reversible half-ring traction leg splint (Keller-Blake)

    1 hand towel with 10 spring clips (or large safety pins)

    9 yd. of traction cord

    3 weight carriers and 15 pounds of weights

    2 5½ ft. upright posts each with a swivel end clamp and an upper and lower toggle clamp

    1 8 ft. plain tube

    2 18-in. traction arms with end clamps

    1 9-in. traction arm with end clamp

    7 pulleys with clamp assemblies

    1 trapeze with clamp and hook

    2 6-in. shock blocks

This arrangement is useful in the treatment of fractures of the shaft of the femur in children who are too old for Bryant's traction but young enough that extension of the knee does not angulate the fracture. A skin traction arrangement such as illustrated in Figure 17 is a simpler alternative but lacks the advantages of floating traction. Skeletal traction arrangements such as shown in Figures 31 and 40 are also satisfactory alternatives but are unpopular with many surgeons because of the possibility of pin tract complications.

The skin traction is applied as described previously. Due regard must be given to the possibility of circulatory inadequacy. The limb rests on a pad consisting of a stockinette covered strip of sponge or saddler's felt. The pad in turn rests on a hammock consisting of towels or canvas straps pinned tightly between the side bars of the traction splint. The Keller-Blake splint, having a hinged half-ring, is superior to the full-ring Thomas splint. The half-rings and straps of newer models are padded and covered by the manufacturer with waterproof plastic, which facilitates cleaning and eliminates the need for additional padding. The half-ring should be oriented anteriorly to facilitate personal hygiene and to prevent it from pushing the proximal fragment of the femur into greater flexion. If the half-ring tends to rest on the groin, it may be necessary to tie the ring in acute anteflexion. DiCosola rope holders mounted on the side bars serve as handy fixation points for this purpose and also prevent the suspension cords from sliding up the side bars. See Figure 33. The modified half-ring splint, with an adjustable offset in the medial bar, developed by Ilfeld, would seem to obviate these difficulties.

Just enough counterweight should be attached to the cords supporting each end of the splint to float the splint and leg and to allow the child to lift himself onto the bedpan without disturbing the fracture. Regardless of how the suspension cords are attached to the splint, some children will manage to capsize it. If such tendencies can be anticipated, it is wise to wrap an elastic bandage about the entire leg and splint. To prevent the child from pushing the splint off the leg, the main traction cord should be tied to the narrow end of the splint enroute from spreader to pulley. Shock blocks must be used beneath the foot of the bed to provide countertraction. The child may turn as he wishes from the waist up but should not turn his pelvis. In actual practice children usually remain quiet and cooperative until enough union has occurred that movement in bed is no longer hazardous. When the child regains his normal hyperactivity and the fracture site is no longer tender to palpation, x-ray examination will usually reveal sufficiently mature callus to justify removal of the traction, application of a spica cast and discharge from the hospital.

References

Ilfeld, F. W.: A modified half-ring splint and combined foot support and exerciser. J. Bone & Joint Surg., *43A:*139, 1961.
Conwell, H. E.: Acute fractures of the shaft of the femur in children. J. Bone & Joint Surg., *11:*593, 1929.

Skin Traction on the Lower Leg with Separate Skin Traction on the Thigh for a Proximal Shaft Fracture of the Femur

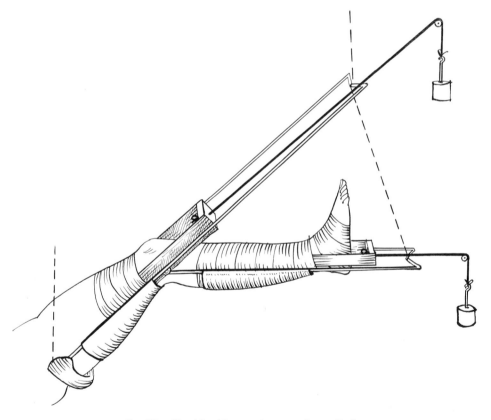

Fig. 19.   Double skin traction on a lower limb.

This arrangement is mentioned only for completeness. Its use is not recommended. If the elastic bandage about the thigh is wrapped snugly enough for the traction tape to stay in place under even light loads, the venous and lymphatic return is usually compromised. If wrapped loosely, or if inadequate traction loads are applied, the entire dressing is likely to slip, compressing the popliteal space. Furthermore, very little skin of the thigh is actually available for traction since, for effective pull, the tape cannot extend proximal to the level of the fracture. In general, the conditions for which this traction arrangement was designed can be better treated by some other method. See Figures 17, 18, 31 and 40.

Dunlop's Traction for Transcondylar and Supracondylar Fractures of the Humerus in Children

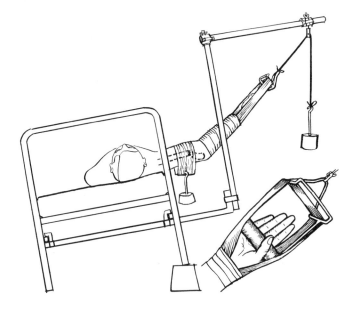

Fig. 20.   Dunlop's traction by a frame attaching under the bed.

Equipment

    1 strip of commercial sponge traction tape or 1 long strip of moleskin or 3 long strips of 2-in. adhesive tape
    1 3-in. elastic bandage
    1 wire spreader with hand grip
    1 yd. of traction cord
    1 stockinette covered felt sling 3 in. wide and 12 in. long (Figure 15)
    2 weight carriers and 10 pounds of weights
    1 base clamp assembly which can be fastened to the undercarriage of the bed
    1 36-in. traction arm with end clamp
    1 27-in. traction arm with end clamp
    1 pulley with clamp assembly
    2 6-in. shock blocks
    1 body restraint

Dunlop's traction is an extremely useful means of handling those transcondylar and supracondylar fractures of the humerus in children in which closed reduction cannot be performed easily or in which elbow flexion is likely to compromise circulation to the hand. Even with the elbow extended in Dunlop's traction, it is essential that the circulation in the hand be checked frequently to avoid the disabling complication of Volkmann's contracture.

Satisfactory Dunlop's traction can be obtained with a number of different devices or pipe arrangements which either rest independently on the floor or attach directly to the bed. The latter system is somewhat safer and permits moving the bed on the ward. The arrangement depicted in Figure 20 is quite simple but requires a special base clamp assembly to secure the arm-supporting poles to the bed.

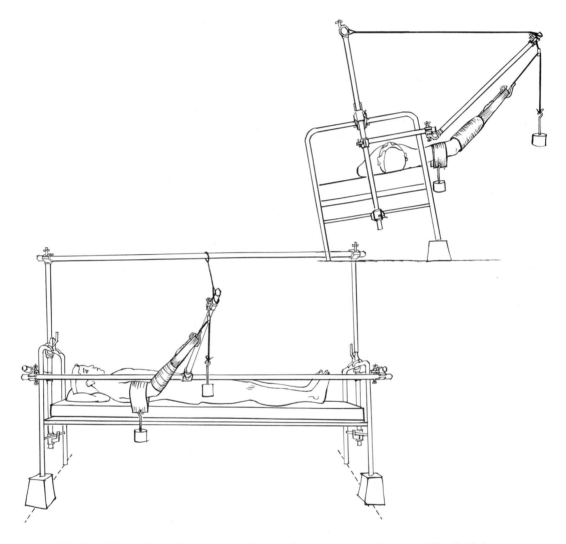

Fig. 21. Dunlop's traction using double swivel clamps to permit upward tilt of side bar.

Equipment

        1 strip of commercial sponge traction tape or 1 long strip of moleskin or 3 long strips of 2-in. adhesive tape

        1 3-in. elastic bandage

        1 wire spreader with hand grip (Fig. 20)

        2 yd. of traction cord

        1 stockinette covered felt sling 3 in. wide and 12 in. long (Fig. 15)

        2 weight carriers and 10 pounds of weights

        2 5½ ft. upright posts each with a swivel end clamp and an upper and lower toggle clamp

        2 18-in. traction arms with end clamps

2 double swivel clamps
2 8 ft. plain tubes
1 27-in. traction arm with end clamp
1 pulley with clamp assembly
1 body restraint

The arrangement depicted in Figure 21 involves more equipment than usually used in Dunlop's traction but has the advantage of permitting passage of the bed through doorways to and from the anesthesia room with minimal disturbance. Double swivel clamps or, if these are not available, traction cord lashings are used at each end of the long longitudinal lateral poles. Either form of attachment permits sufficient motion to allow the outermost crossbar to be pushed upward easily. A piece of traction cord to the overhead pole serves as a checkrein to prevent too much depression of this crossbar.

Regardless of the arrangement used, the extremity should be maintained with the elbow at about 135° with an outward and upward pull on the forearm and a light downward pull on the apex of the anteriorly angulated humeral fragments. The patient must be kept constantly at the edge of the bed. Shock blocks under the traction side of the bed, a vest type restraint, and a bed side through or under which the arm is threaded serve to maintain this position. When a bed side is used in this fashion, it is wise to secure it by adhesive tape or other means to prevent its being lowered carelessly. In the arrangement depicted in Figure 21, the long longitudinal lateral pole substitutes for the bed side.

The adhesive tape or other skin traction device is applied to the forearm as already described for the leg on page 13. A small space should be left between the wrappings of the elastic bandage on the volar aspect for palpation of the radial pulse. The tape should extend proximally to the antecubital flexor crease but should not cover the olecranon. If the skin over the olecranon is left undisturbed and skin traction proves inadequate, skeletal traction may then be applied through this area. See Figure 43.

A wire spreader with an attached hand grip for use with Dunlop's traction is now on the market. If it is not available, one can be improvised by strapping together several tongue blades and tying or strapping them to an ordinary spreader. Such a device enhances the patient's comfort by promoting use of the fingers and relieving some of the tension from the skin.

The traction is adjusted to suspend the extremity with sufficient elevation that the edge of the mattress does not tend to push the proximal fragment of the humerus upward. The forearm should preferably lie in supination.

The sling is made by slipping a 3-in. wide, 1 ft. long strip of ½-in. thick saddler's felt into a stockinette tube and is used with a 2 or 3 pound weight. This sling should be maintained over the distal end of the proximal fragment.

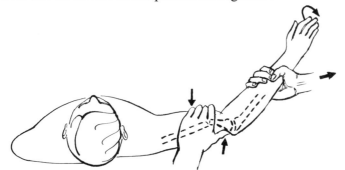

Fig. 22.   Manipulative reduction of supracondylar fracture.

During or after application of the traction, manual reduction of the fracture may be performed by increasing the traction with one hand while pushing upward on the distal fragment of the humerus and the olecranon with the thumb of the other hand. After swelling has subsided, reduction has been obtained, and some degree of union is revealed by the radiologic appearance of callus, the elbow may be brought gradually into increasing flexion by moving the supporting pulley inward on the overarm bar. When flexion greater than 90° has been achieved without loss of position, a long arm cast may then be applied and secured with a collar and cuff sling and swathe. With this protection the child may be sent home for the remainder of his convalescence.

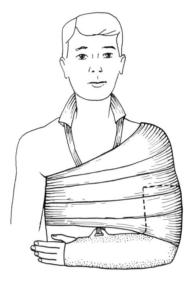

Fig. 23.   Post-traction immobilization with hanging cast and swathe.

References

Caldwell, J. A.: Treatment of fracture of the shaft of the humerus by hanging cast. Surg. Gynec. & Obst., *70:*421, 1940.
Dunlop, J.: Transcondylar fractures of the humerus in children. J. Bone & Joint Surg., *21:*59, 1939.
Griffiths, D. L.: Volkmann's ischaemic contracture. Brit. J. Surg., *28:*239, 1940.

Skin Traction on the Forearm with Separate Skin Traction on the Upper Arm for a Fracture of the Clavicle or Proximal Humerus

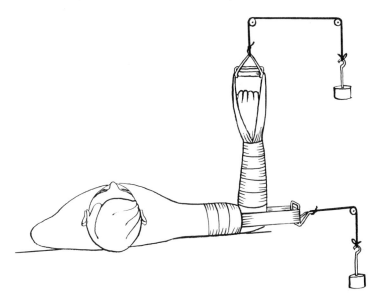

Fig. 24.   Double skin traction on an upper limb.

Equipment

   2 strips of commercial sponge traction tape or 2 long strips of moleskin or 4 long strips of 2-in. adhesive tape
   2 3-in. elastic bandages
   1 wire spreader with hand grip (Fig. 20)
   1 small spreader block
   2 yd. of traction cord
   2 weight carriers and 10 pounds of weights
   1 base clamp assembly which can be fastened to the undercarriage of the bed (Fig. 43)
   1 36-in. traction arm with end clamp
   1 27-in. traction arm with end clamp
   1 9-in. traction arm with end clamp
   3 pulleys with clamp assemblies
   2 6-in. shock blocks

Skin traction on the upper arm is less than ideal owing to the limited skin surface available for attachment of the tape and the consequent tendency of both tape and overlying elastic bandage to slip distally, constricting the antecubital space. If, in order to secure better purchase of the tape on the skin, the elastic bandage is wrapped tightly, distal swelling will occur. For these reasons, only light traction loads can be used and the arrangement must be inspected frequently. Since the tape must not extend proximal to the level of the fracture, there is too little skin on the upper arm available for attachment of the tape if the fracture is below the proximal quarter of the shaft. Hence this type of traction is of value only with certain fractures of the clavicle and certain subtubercular fractures of the humerus. With clavicular fractures, it is worthwhile only when an optimal cosmetic result is necessary, as with a debutante or female night club singer. With subtubercular fractures, it should be used only when other methods of treatment are contraindicated or unsuccessful, as when general anesthesia for manipulative reduction is contraindicated, when manipulation fails, when the patient cannot be kept erect so that a hanging cast can be used, or when skeletal traction (Fig. 43) is not desired or is contraindicated because of wounds about the elbow.

To achieve effective traction on a fractured clavicle, a pad must be maintained between the shoulder blades, allowing the shoulders to drop backwards. With a sub-tubercular fracture of the humerus, such a pad must not be used, and the patient must be kept in the center of the bed so that the mattress supports the upper arm. In either case low shock blocks are placed under the traction side of the bed. The buttocks may be lifted for the bedpan. A patient with a fracture of the humerus may roll slightly toward the involved side for back care. One with a fracture of the clavicle may roll slightly toward the opposite side. Otherwise, these patients must be kept flat.

Reference

Blount, W. P.: Fractures in Children. Baltimore, Williams and Wilkins Company, 1955.

SKELETAL TRACTION

Special Features

Skeletal traction, achieved by inserting a metal device directly into the bone, withstands very high forces for prolonged periods of time and is, therefore, the most reliable means of securing an effective traction force. Various types of hooks, tongs, screws, pins, and wires have been used for this purpose. In most cases either a Kirschner wire or a Steinmann pin is eminently satisfactory. Of these two, the Kirschner wire, with its smaller diameter, makes a smaller wound and causes less discomfort to the patient.

The duration of use of these devices is limited only by the development of sepsis in the tract through the bone. Such a complication is almost inevitable if the wire remains *in situ* for 3 or 4 months. Such an infection usually subsides spontaneously upon removal of the wire. Rarely it may not subside and may prove troublesome, particularly in children, in whom it may involve the nearby epiphyseal plate and provoke a local growth disturbance.

Additional difficulties attendant upon the use of traction devices in long bones may be largely avoided by proper placement in the correct metaphysis. Transfixion of a diaphysis should be avoided. Such a practice will occasionally lead to a fracture through the pin tract after function is resumed. The pin or wire should pass through a minimum of sliding soft tissues. Infraction of this rule leads to stiffness in adjacent joints. This problem renders the use of skeletal traction in fractures of the hand of doubtful value compared with accurate open reduction and internal fixation. Whenever possible, fracture hematomas should not be violated. This is seldom necessary except in the treatment of calcaneal fractures by traction. Finally, for the most efficient traction, the metaphysis closest to the fracture should be the one selected for transfixion provided the above conditions are satisfied. Thus, for a tibial plateau fracture, the distal tibial metaphysis is used. For a low femoral shaft fracture, the proximal tibial metaphysis is preferred. With subtrochanteric fractures, the distal femoral metaphysis should be used.

Pain at the traction site beyond a few days after application is usually an indication that either there is a pin tract infection or the wire is not actually in the bone and is therefore pulling on soft tissue. The latter circumstance is usually caused by incorrect initial insertion of the wire. It is exceedingly uncommon for a properly placed traction wire to migrate in bone.

Insertion of Kirschner Wires and Steinmann Pins

In order to minimize the chances of infection, skeletal traction should be applied under strictly sterile conditions with proper surgical skin preparation and draping. Satisfactory conditions may be available in the emergency department or a treatment room, but the ideal location is usually the operating room. Regardless of where the procedure is performed, a previously sterilized kit facilitates the matter.

Kirschner Wire Insertion Tray

> Prep. solution cups
> Prep. sponge clamps
> Sponges
> Draping towels
> Towel clips
> Hypodermic needle and syringe
> Assorted Kirschner wires
> Assorted sizes of Kirschner wire tractor bows
> Cannulated hand drill with chuck key
> Heavy pliers with a wire-cutting throat

If Steinmann pins are included, a Bohler-Steinmann pin bow and a large double action pin cutter are needed.

After the site of insertion has been chosen and the area prepped and draped, the point of insertion and a tract down to the bone are anesthetized. If a small nick is made through the skin, insertion of the wire causes less puckering and is less painful but is somewhat more likely to lead to a pin tract infection. Because of the flexibility of a Kirschner wire, it must be mounted in a cannulated drill with only a couple of inches protruding. Such a hand drill is far more satisfactory than the older Kirschner wire drills with outriggers. The wire should always be inserted in a plane perpendicular to the anticipated line of traction. This plane is approximately perpendicular to the longitudinal axis of the bone. In the case of a fractured femur, one may correct rotation by inserting the pin somewhat obliquely within this plane rather than horizontally, recognizing that if the ends of the wire are left long enough they will come to rest on the side bars of the traction splint and in so doing impart a certain amount of torque to the distal fragment. After the wire has been pushed through the soft tissues, it is spun through the bone and through the soft tissue on the opposite side. The amount of wire protruding from the hand drill is lengthened as needed. Local infiltration of the soft tissues ahead of the wire as it emerges renders the entire procedure almost painless. The wire is driven until equal lengths protrude from both sides of the limb. Dressings are most likely to stay in place if threaded over the ends of the wire prior to attachment of the bow. If slightly bulky dressings are used and then compressed by the use of the narrowest bow that will fit, sideways slip of the wire is minimized. Threaded wires are also a help in this respect, but in the author's experience they are likely to break under heavy loads. The handle of the Kirschner wire tractor bow should, of course, be twisted as tightly as possible to minimize bowing of the wires. If correction of rotation is not needed, the ends of the wire may be bent up along the arms of the bow and strapped to them with adhesive tape. This refinement protects the bed linen and the patient's opposite extremity, and locks the wire clamps on the ends of the bow. It is superior to impaling corks on the wire tips.

Experience has shown the necessity for warning interns or assistant residents who may be learning to insert Kirschner wires or Steinmann pins, that a Kirschner wire tractor will not work satisfactorily with a Steinmann pin nor a Steinmann pin bow with a Kirschner wire. The new Salvatore nylon disposable bow is an exception; it will accommodate to both wires and pins.

Reference

Steinmann, F.: Zur Geschichte der Nagelextension. Zeitschr. Orth. Chir., *29:*96, 1911.

Through Calcaneus for Fracture of Calcaneus with Loss of Tuber-joint Angle

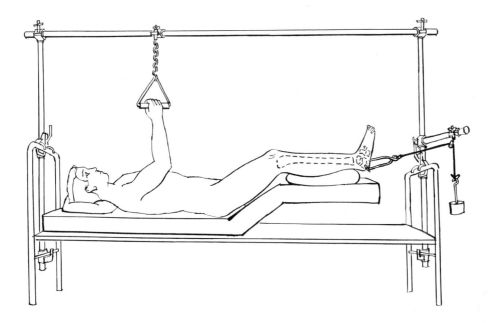

Fig. 25. Calcaneal traction with flexed knee for calcaneal fracture.

Equipment

 1 Kirschner wire or Steinmann pin insertion tray
 1 yd. of traction cord
 1 weight carrier and 10 pounds of weights
 2 5½ ft. upright posts each with a swivel end clamp and an upper and lower toggle clamp
 1 18-in. traction arm with end clamp
 1 pulley with clamp assembly
 1 8-ft. plain tube
 1 trapeze with clamp and hook
 1 large pillow
 2 6-in. shock blocks

Although treatment of a fracture of the calcaneus by traction is uncommon and presents the disadvantage of contamination of the fracture hematoma by a percutaneous pin, this form of treatment is occasionally useful with a marked loss of the tuber-joint (Bohler's) angle, particularly in a foot that is swelling rapidly. After the pin is inserted the fracture should be reduced by manual traction on the Steinmann pin bow. The pulley and weight traction is then used merely to maintain reduction without the danger of compression by a plaster cast. A Steinmann pin is sometimes preferred to a Kirschner wire in this circumstance since, because of its larger caliber, it is perhaps less likely to migrate through the soft fractured cancellous bone.

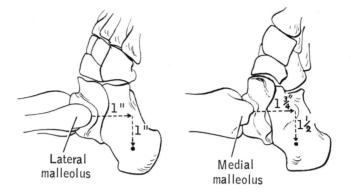

Fig. 26. Preferred site for insertion of traction pin through the calcaneus.

The correct spot for insertion of the pin may be measured from the malleoli, these being landmarks which can be palpated in very swollen feet. Ideally, the pin should be inserted as far posterior as possible while still engaging sound bone. The tendons and neurovascular bundle passing behind the malleoli, and, of course, the talocalcaneal joint are to be avoided. Although in some communities the pin is intentionally placed through the soft tissue space between the talus, calcaneus and tendo achillis, this practice should be abandoned as it leads all too commonly to disastrous slough and infection.

In this injury the lower extremity should be elevated by cranking up the springs and mattress as indicated in Figure 25. If elevation is adequate, shock blocks are sometimes unnecessary, since countertraction is provided by the friction of the thigh against the slanting portion of the mattress. The lower leg must also rest on a soft pillow in such a way as to prevent any friction on the heel. Considerable movement of the patient in bed may be permitted and the back rest may be elevated intermittently provided it does not make the patient slide down in bed and provided the swelling in the foot is subsiding satisfactorily.

References

Bohler, L.: Diagnosis, pathology and treatment of fractures of os calcis. J. Bone & Joint Surg., *13:*75, 1931.
Schofield, R. O.: Fractures of the os calcis, J. Bone & Joint Surg., *18:*566, 1936.

Through Calcaneus for Extensive Open Fracture of the Tibia and Fibula

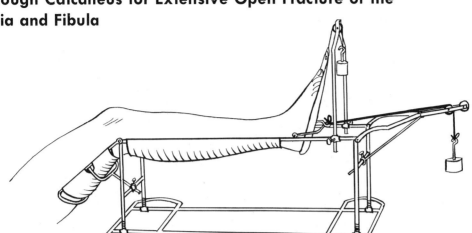

Fig. 27.   Bohler-Braun frame with skeletal traction on the calcaneus and skin traction on the forefoot.

Equipment

     1 Kirschner wire or Steinmann pin insertion tray
     1 yd. of traction cord
     2 weight carriers and 10 pounds of weights
     1 Bohler-Braun frame

Traction is occasionally useful in the immobilization of an open fracture of the tibia and fibula with extensive loss of soft tissue, when need for frequent wound care makes a complete plaster cast undesirable. Under such circumstances almost any major movement of the patient's trunk is likely to cause undesirable motion at the fracture site. For this reason one should use a fracture bed with a built-in Bradford frame and depressible mattress by virtue of which the bedpan may be placed under the patient with minimal disturbance. The injured limb must be supported with the hip and knee in moderate flexion. This position may be achieved by placing the limb in an appropriately counterbalanced posterior plaster shell as advocated by Urist, or by placing it in a Keller-Blake splint and Pearson attachment suspended as illustrated in Figure 31. This position may also be obtained by use of a Bohler-Braun frame. The patient immobilized in such a frame must remain even quieter than in a suspension system if he is not to disturb his fracture. On the other hand, the Bohler-Braun frame is much simpler to apply, and it provides adequate support and immobilization in most of these fractures until the soft tissues have healed and the limb may be placed in a long leg cast. Shock blocks are seldom necessary if the frame is adjusted so that the thigh rests against the frame at a fairly high angle. Equinus is prevented by attaching a wide strip of adhesive tape to the sole of the foot and applying a light traction force to this tape in an upward direction. This precaution is particularly important with concurrent anterior compartment muscle injuries or peroneal nerve palsies. The correct location for placement of the calcaneal traction pin is shown in Figure 26.

Reference

Urist, M. R., Ries, L., Quigley, T. B.: A plaster traction splint for compound comminuted fractures of tibia and fibula. Surgery, *23*:801, 1948.

Through Calcaneus or Distal Tibia and Fibula for
Increased Traction on a Fractured Hip

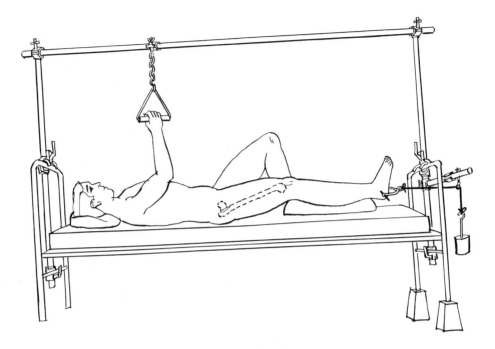

Fig. 28.   Calcaneal traction with knee extended.

Equipment

       1 Kirschner wire or Steinmann pin insertion tray
       1 yd. of traction cord
       1 weight carrier and 15 pounds of weights
       2 5½ ft. upright posts each with a swivel end clamp and an upper and lower toggle clamp
       1 18-in. traction arm with end clamp
       1 pulley with clamp assembly
       1 8 ft. plain tube
       1 trapeze with clamp and hook
       1 large pillow
       2 10-in. shock blocks

When the distal femoral fragment of a broken hip has migrated proximally and become somewhat fixed in this position by contracted soft tissues, greater traction force may be necessary in order to stretch out these tissues than can be achieved with Buck's skin traction. In such cases the desired effect may be obtained by skeletal traction applied to the calcaneus or to the distal tibia and fibula. The knee and hip should be kept in relative extension, with only a single pillow used under the lower leg to reduce friction of the heel against the mattress and to permit transmission of the force to the region of the hip. Countertraction is obtained by elevation of the foot of the bed on shock blocks. Neither the back rest nor the knee rest should be elevated.

Landmarks for insertion of the traction pin through the calcaneus are shown in Figure 26 and for insertion through the distal tibia and fibula in Figure 30.

Through Distal Tibia and Fibula for Tibial Plateau Fracture

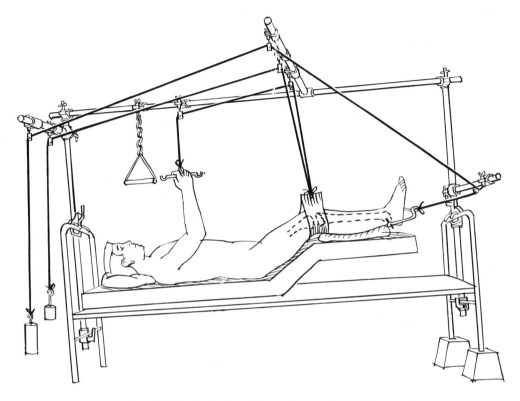

Fig. 29.   Skeletal split Russell's traction with exercising cord.

Equipment

 1 Kirschner wire or Steinmann pin insertion tray
 1 stockinette covered felt sling 4 in. wide and 18 in. long (Fig. 15)
 9 yd. of traction cord
 2 weight carriers and 20 pounds of weights
 1 6-in. spreader bar for use as an exercising handle
 2 5½ ft. upright posts each with a swivel end clamp and an upper and lower toggle clamp
 1 8 ft. plain tube
 3 18-in. traction arms with end clamps
 7 pulleys with clamp assemblies
 1 trapeze with clamp and hook
 1 large pillow
 2 6-in. shock blocks

Properly applied traction for tibial plateau fractures has been found extremely useful in the treatment of certain of these rather disabling injuries. When a few large fragments are present, open reduction with screw or bolt fixation may be the ideal treatment. If fixation is thought not to be absolutely secure following such a procedure, the operation may then be followed by either light traction or a plaster cast. If, on the other hand, the fragments are too small and numerous to permit exact repositioning by surgery, the initial use of traction offers certain advantages to casting. By maintaining the limb in partial hip and knee flexion with appropriate elevation of the mattress, and by applying a moderately heavy traction load to a pin inserted through the distal tibia and fibula, impaction forces on the knee can be reduced sufficiently to facilitate manipulative reduction. With the patient under anesthesia, the surgeon can then mold the plateau by interlacing his fingers behind the knee and forcefully compressing the sides of the proximal tibia with the heels of his hands. Aspiration of the hemarthrosis may be necessary. A stockinette covered felt sling around the fracture, pulling upward, also helps in molding and maintaining position. In view of the magnitude and direction of the main traction force, shock blocks under the foot of the bed are usually necessary. Within a couple of weeks after the injury knee flexion and extension exercises must be initiated in order to achieve a good range of motion. With an exercising cord attached to the sling and run through an overhead pulley to a handle within reach, the patient can assist himself in these exercises.

Before inserting the pin, one should check to see if the tractor bow is of adequate size to avoid pressure on the sole of the foot when attached to the pin. The arms of Bohler-Steinmann pin bows may usually be bent in such a way as to increase their effective length. Since this is not true of Kirschner wire tractors, and since, with an adult male patient, the largest Kirschner wire tractors are sometimes not long enough, one may prefer to use a Steinmann pin rather than a Kirschner wire.

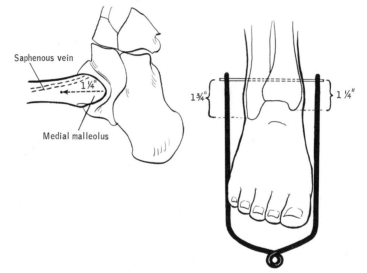

Fig. 30. Preferred site for insertion of traction pin through the distal tibia and fibula.

The pin should pass through the center of the lateral surface of the fibula, thereby avoiding injury to the peroneal tendon sheaths, and through the center of the medial surface of the tibia, thereby avoiding the extensor tendons and neurovascular bundle entering the tarsal tunnel posteriorly. If the pin is inserted 2 in. proximal to the tip of the medial malleolus, the tibiotalar joint will be avoided. Finally, care should be taken to miss the saphenous vein.

Reference

Apley, A. G.: Fractures of the lateral tibial condyle treated by skeletal traction and early mobilization. A review of sixty cases with special reference to the long-term results. J. Bone & Joint Surg., *38B*:699, 1956.

Through Proximal Tibia for Fracture of the Distal Two-Thirds of the Femur: Balanced Suspension

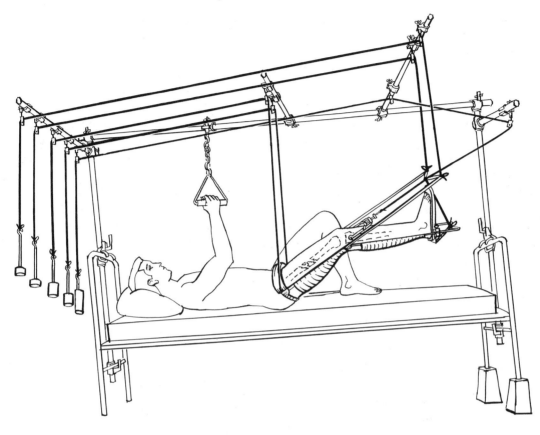

Fig. 31. Proximal tibial traction with balanced suspension.

Equipment

- 1 Kirschner wire insertion tray
- 1 reversible half-ring traction leg splint (Keller-Blake)
- 1 Pearson attachment
- 2 hand towels with 12 spring clips (or large safety pins)
- 1 elastic activated foot plate
- 18 yd. of traction cord
- 5 weight carriers and 35 pounds of weights
- 2 5½ ft. upright posts each with a swivel end clamp and an upper and lower toggle clamp
- 1 8-ft. plain tube
- 4 18-in. traction arms with end clamps
- 10 pulleys with clamp assemblies
- 1 trapeze with clamp and hook
- 2 10-in. shock blocks

This arrangement, of great value in the treatment of fractures of the distal two-thirds of the shaft of the femur in older children and adults, consists of two separate but related systems. One, a traction system, consists of a skeletal wire or pin, the tractor bow and its attached traction line, a crossbar and pulley at the foot of the bed, and a heavy weight. The patient is kept from sliding under the influence of this traction force by elevation of the foot of the bed on high shock blocks. Neither the back rest nor the knee rest of the bed can be elevated without interfering with the equilibrium of traction and countertraction forces. The other system, known as balanced suspension, is designed to float the lower limb in such a way as to prevent angulation forces at the fracture site as the patient moves vertically in bed in the process of getting on and off the bedpan. This latter system consists of a "traction" splint, Pearson attachment, supporting towels or slings, 4 suspending cords, 2 overhead crossbars with pulleys, and 4 small counterbalancing weights.

Both the traction and suspension systems are arranged somewhat differently, depending upon the level of the fracture. In general, the more proximal the fracture, the more the proximal fragment is flexed anteriorly by the iliopsoas muscle. For this reason, when the fracture is located in the upper third of the shaft, it is usually necessary to orient the longitudinal axis of the distal fragment vertically in order to align it with the sharply flexed proximal fragment. This orientation is best obtained with 90–90 traction as shown in Figure 40. In general, the more distal the fracture, the less the proximal fragment is flexed anteriorly and the more the distal fragment is flexed posteriorly by the gastrocnemius muscle. For this reason, when the fracture is located in the lower third or supracondylar area, the thigh need not be supported at a very high angle but the knee should be flexed more sharply. The Pearson attachment should be fastened to the side bars of the traction splint at the level of the fracture rather than the knee joint, thereby creating a fulcrum around which the limb can be pulled to help correct alignment. Orientation of the main traction cord at a downward angle with respect to the longitudinal axis of the thigh is also helpful in this regard. See Figure 35. On the other hand, when the fracture lies in the middle third of the femur, a better balance of muscle pull on the bone fragments prevails. In this case the thigh should be supported at approximately 40° of hip flexion, and the main traction cord should be aligned with the longitudinal axis of the thigh. This cord will then lie in contact with the transverse part of the small end of the traction splint. See Figure 36.

Assembly of the apparatus and attachment of the patient in this arrangement are facilitated by following the steps in sequence as described below. Careful attention to detail is rewarding in terms of patient comfort and time spent in later adjustment.

A traction splint of adequate length, breadth and design is selected. Keller-Blake splints having hinged half-rings may be reversed for use with either leg, are readily stored, and are superior for present purposes to the older full-ring variety of Thomas splint. Ilfeld's splint, distinguished by a right-angled offset in the proximal part of the medial bar, would seem to fit still better. If the half-ring is properly covered with neoprene or similar waterproof material by the manufacturer, additional padding is unnecessary and untidy. A Pearson attachment is clamped to the sides of the traction splint, at the level where the fracture will lie in the case of supracondylar fractures, or at the level of the femoral condyles in the case of mid-shaft fractures. The proximal portions of the splint and Pearson attachment are spanned with small hand towels pinned about each rod. These should be stretched tightly except near the half-ring, where considerable sag should be permitted to accommodate the bulk of the proximal thigh. Commercial straps and clips are easier to use than towels but are usually not available at the right time and place. A felt or sponge pad placed on top of the towels will greatly enhance patient comfort. It should extend from proximal thigh to heel, be of ½-in. thickness and cut almost as wide as the splint. Prior to placing this pad on the splint, it should be slipped into a stockinette sleeve.

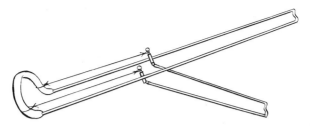

Fig. 32. Anteflexion of the half-ring maintained by tying the sides of the half-ring to the screw clamps of the Pearson attachment. When the thigh is small, a single cord tied tightly between the half-ring and the narrow end of the splint suffices.

The half-ring of the Keller-Blake splint is then turned upward so that it will ultimately lie over the groin rather than posteriorly against the ischial tuberosity. The anterior position is preferred in balanced suspension because it facilitates use of the bedpan and does not promote undesirable flexion of the hip. Furthermore, counter-traction is obtained by tilting the bed with shock blocks rather than by impingement of the ring on the ischial tuberosity as in Figure 2. Frequently the half-ring tends to drop down spontaneously, thereby irritating the skin over the anterior superior spine of the ilium. This tendency can be prevented by tying two pieces of traction cord from the sides of the half-ring to the screw clamps of the Pearson attachment, or, if the thigh is thin, by tying a single cord from the center of the half-ring to the opposite end of the splint.

After the supporting splint has been dressed as described and placed on the bed, the overhead frame with appropriate crossbars and pulleys is assembled as illustrated in Figure 31. The two crossbars intended to support the splint and leg should be placed directly above each end of the splint. In the case of a mid-shaft fracture, the crossbar for the main traction line should be clamped either to the very top of the 5½ ft. upright pole or close by on the foot end of the 8-ft. longitudinal pole. In the case of a supra-condylar fracture, this crossbar should be clamped somewhat lower on the 5½ ft. up-right pole. A final crossbar with 5 pulleys is attached to the overhead frame at the head end of the bed to carry all traction cords to this end, where the weights will hang freely when the foot of the bed is elevated on shock blocks and where the weights will not be disturbed by passers-by.

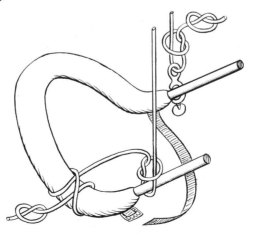

Fig. 33. Alternate techniques for attachment of the 2 suspension cords at the proximal end of the traction splint, to prevent distal slip of the cords along the side bars. DiCosola rope holder with slip knot at top; slip knot and clove-hitch at bottom.

After assembly of the overhead frame, supporting cords are attached to the splint and run through the pulleys as indicated. Although a single cord running from each end of the splint will suffice, the use of a cord from each corner provides more precise control of rotation and is preferable if sufficient equipment is available. In attaching the suspension cords to the proximal end of the splint, care must be taken to tie them in such a way that they cannot slip upward along the smooth side bars. DiCosola rope holders are helpful, or the cord may be tied about both side bars and half-ring.

After the distal ends of the traction splint and the Pearson attachment are connected by a short piece of cord, the main traction line is run through its pulleys and the ends of this cord are left in readiness for later attachment to the Kirschner wire tractor bow and the main traction weight.

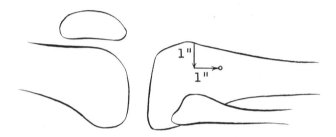

Fig. 34.   Preferred site for insertion of traction wire through the proximal tibia.

After proper skin preparation and local infiltration, the Kirschner wire should be passed transversely through the proximal tibial metaphysis, avoiding the proximal epiphyseal plate cephalad, the epiphyseal plate of the tibial tubercle anteriorly, and the branches of the peroneal nerve posteriorly. Furthermore, the wire should not pass through the cortical bone of the proximal diaphysis, particularly the anterior crest of the tibia, since the pin tract weakens that structure and thus occasionally leads to fractures after ambulation is resumed. The ideal location of this wire, therefore, is approximately 1 in. posterior to the tibial tubercle and 1 in. distal to it in the average adult.

After application of dressings about the Kirschner wire and attachment of the tractor bow, the patient can be transferred from the stretcher to the bed. The injured extremity is lifted gently by pulling distally and upwards on the bow while supporting the lower leg. The traction splint with Pearson attachment, towels, pad, and supporting cords is then slipped into place. The main traction line is then tied securely to the tractor bow and the necessary weight (from 15 to 30 pounds) is attached to the opposite end of this line. Adequate weights to float the splint and leg are attached to the free ends of the 4 supporting cords. When the assembly is properly adjusted and balanced, the half-ring does not press on the skin.

If precautions are not taken soon after the patient is placed in balanced suspension, the splint may gradually slip distally on the leg. With a supracondylar fracture this difficulty is prevented by tying a piece of cord under slight tension from the narrow end of the splint to the Kirschner wire bow. With a mid-shaft fracture the problem is solved simply by tying the main traction line and the transverse part of the splint securely together where they cross.

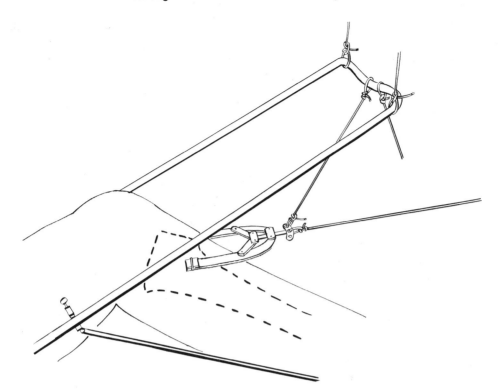

Fig. 35.   In supracondylar fracture, distal displacement of splint prevented by a cord from splint to bow. Note lower angle of splint, greater knee flexion, and proximal connection of Pearson attachment.

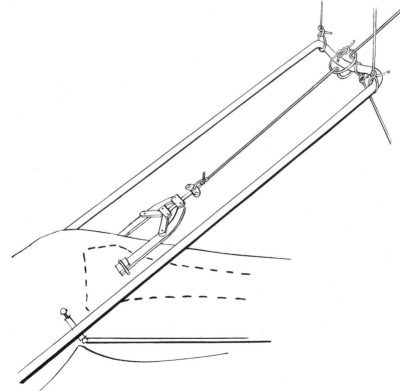

Fig. 36.   In mid-shaft fracture, displacement of splint prevented by tying main traction line and splint together. Note higher angle of splint, reduced knee flexion, and more distal connection of Pearson attachment.

Finally, a spring or elastic activated foot plate may be attached to the Pearson attachment to protect the power of the foot dorsiflexors. Although important with adults, this refinement is seldom necessary with children unless a neurologic defect is present.

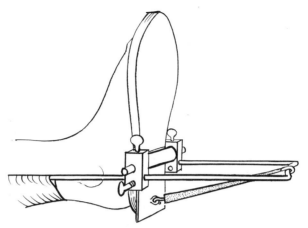

Fig. 37.   Elastic activated foot plate.

During convalescence, clinical and radiologic examinations will reveal the need for various adjustments. Alterations of the amount of weight on the main traction line and other cords are usually necessary at different stages of reduction. Occasionally it is necessary to insert a small folded sheet or towel at the proper point under the thigh to restore the normal anterior bow of the femur. If the fragments are displaced in the coronal plane, movement of the pulleys toward or away from the mid-line is helpful in restoring alignment. An observation of weak foot dorsiflexion or a complaint of pain distal to the tibial traction wire should direct immediate attention to the soft tissues behind the fibular head. A common cause of pressure on the peroneal nerve at this point is distal slip of the splint or Pearson attachment.

It should be appreciated that by pulling on the trapeze and pressing on the mattress with the uninjured limb, the patient may move himself vertically and longitudinally. Assistance of his movements should, of course, be performed by moving his trunk, not his leg. If shock blocks under the foot of the bed are not high enough, the patient must consciously maintain a position toward the head of the bed. No attempt at turning from the waist down is permissible.

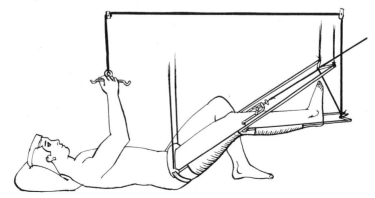

Fig. 38.   Knee exerciser in balanced suspension.

As early evidence of some union is revealed by the loss of tenderness at the fracture site and by the radiologic appearance of immature callus, gentle knee and hip exercises may be initiated. These may be assisted by an exercising cord run from the distal end of the traction splint to overhead pulleys to a handle consisting of a head halter spreader bar or a bundle of tongue blades within the patient's reach.

When the callus appears sufficiently mature and there is no longer motion at the fracture site, it may be elected in the interest of the patient's financial status to remove him gently from the entire traction apparatus and apply a hip spica cast. If the family can care for him in this state, he may then be sent home to await more solid union.

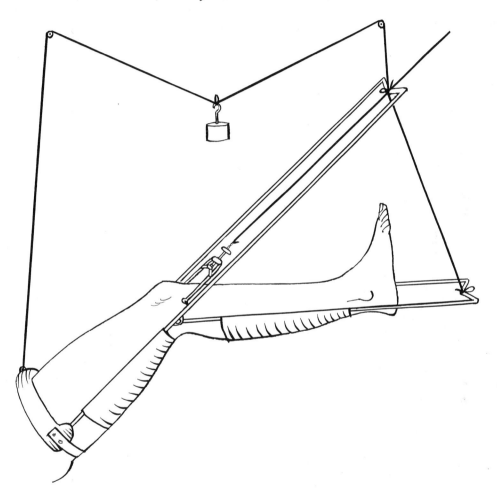

Fig. 39. Balanced suspension by a single weight.

The technique of suspending the traction splint and leg by one continuous cord with 2 overhead pulleys and a single central weight is commonly observed. This practice can be justified only on the basis of inadequate available equipment. The suspended weight usually restricts vertical motion, permits only crude control of the position of the splint and, like the sword of Damocles, constantly threatens the tranquility of the patient.

References

Ilfeld, R. W.: A modified half-ring splint and combined foot support and exerciser. J. Bone & Joint
    Surg., *43A:*139, 1961.
Ritchey, S. J., Schonholtz, G. J., Thompson, M. S.: The dashboard femoral fracture. Pathome-
    chanics, treatment, and prevention. J. Bone & Joint Surg., *40A:*1347, 1958.
Winant, E. M.: The use of skeletal traction in the treatment of fractures of the femur. J. Bone &
    Joint Surg., *31A:*87, 1949.

Through Distal Femur for Subtrochanteric Fracture: 90°–90° Traction

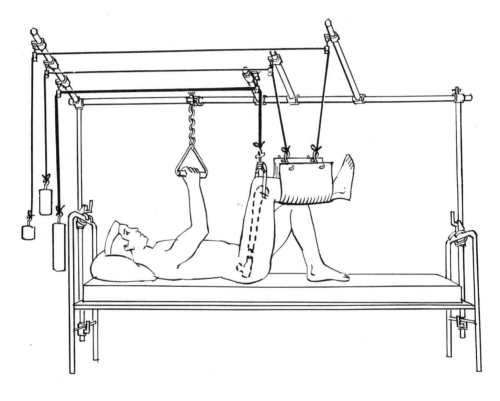

Fig. 40.   90°–90° traction.

Equipment

    1 Kirschner wire or Steinmann pin insertion tray
    1 stockinette covered felt sling 18 by 12 in. (Fig. 15)
 10 yd. of traction cord
    3 weight carriers and 30 pounds of weights
    2 5½ ft. upright posts each with a swivel end clamp and an upper and lower toggle clamp
    1 8 ft. plain tube
    4 18-in. traction arms with end clamps
    6 pulleys with clamp assemblies
    1 trapeze with clamp and hook

Fractures between the lesser trochanter and the junction of the middle and upper thirds of the femur usually present a problem in alignment, owing to sharp flexion of the proximal fragment caused by unopposed pull of the iliopsoas muscle. This problem can usually be solved by inserting a pin across the distal metaphysis and suspending the distal femur vertically over the proximal fragment with traction applied through the pin. The lower leg is supported either by a counterweighted sling or by a Pearson attachment, depending upon local institutional preferences. In this manner the limb is suspended with both knee and hip in 90° of flexion, a position which is fairly comfortable and enables the patient to lift and shift himself slightly by use of the trapeze and his good leg. Of course no turning from the waist down or partial sitting up can be permitted. Although many patients in this situation can manage the bedpan easily, others cannot. Therefore, as with fractures of the pelvis, a fracture bed is helpful. See also Figure 42.

In view of the heavy counterweight (20–30 pounds) needed on the main traction line not only to suspend the thigh but also to overcome muscle pull in aligning the fragments, certain precautions should be taken. One should be particularly certain that all clamps on the overhead frame and crossbars are tightened securely. It is wise to double the main traction line. The proximal tibial metaphysis cannot be used as a traction site because the forces involved cause painful stretching of the knee ligaments. A Kirschner wire should be used only if it is the largest size, i.e. 0.62 in. thick, not threaded or damaged, and securely fastened in a Kirschner wire tractor bow which is tightened forcefully. If a Steinmann pin is used in an adult, it should be ⅛ in. thick. Although smaller sizes may not break, bending becomes a problem.

This traction wire or pin must be inserted with particular care in view of the extent of the suprapatellar pouch anteriorly and proximally, the neurovascular structures behind the distal femur, and, in children, the presence of the distal femoral epiphyseal plate. In general, the pin should pass along or slightly posterior to the mid-coronal plane of the femoral shaft. It should also pass just proximal to the adductor tubercle in order to avoid engagement of the collateral ligaments. When swelling has obscured this landmark, it is helpful to remember that it lies almost at the level of the proximal pole of the patella in the relaxed and extended knee. During actual insertion of the wire, the knee should preferably be flexed in order to draw the periarticular soft tissues into the position they will occupy while the limb is in traction, thereby reducing pressure necrosis.

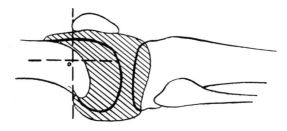

Fig. 41.   Preferred site for insertion of traction pin through the distal femur.

The stockinette covered felt sling in this arrangement has no traction function but serves merely to support and steady the lower leg. This sling should be constructed somewhat wider but in other respects the same as shown in Figure 15. If the overhead pulleys are arranged such that the 2 suspension cords diverge slightly in their course upward, the lower leg is less inclined to pivot when the patient moves. Rotary alignment and, to some extent, abduction and adduction can be controlled by the position of these pulleys with respect to the mid-saggital plane of the patient.

As early evidence of partial union is revealed by loss of tenderness and by radiologic appearance of immature callus, gentle active hip and knee exercises may be initiated. As more union occurs, traction force should be reduced and the traction and suspension pulleys should be moved slowly toward the foot of the bed, thus reducing the degree of hip and knee flexion. Light skin traction applied to the lower leg and pulling toward the foot of the bed is of help in slowly extending the limb. Low shock blocks under the foot of the bed are necessary during this stage. When the thigh has been brought approximately halfway down and if the callus is sufficiently mature, the entire apparatus may be removed as a spica cast is applied. A useful trick at this juncture is to lift the patient vertically in his bed while he is still in traction, slide a spica box or equivalent frame under the patient, and apply the cast while he is still in traction in his bed. The pin can be incorporated in the cast temporarily if desired. There is less chance of angulating the partially united fracture by this technique than by first removing the traction completely and then transferring the patient from his bed to a fracture table. Once in his cast the patient may be sent home for the remainder of the period of immobilization.

Reference

Urist, M. R. and Quigley, T. B.: Use of skeletal traction for mass treatment of compound fractures. A summary of experiences with 4,290 cases during World War II. Arch. Surg., *63*:834, 1951.

Through Proximal Femur for Central Fracture Dislocation of Hip

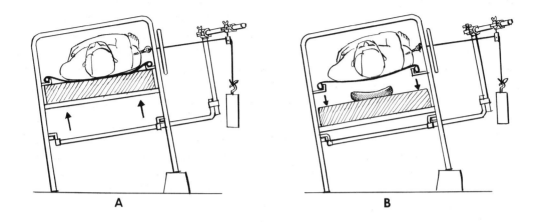

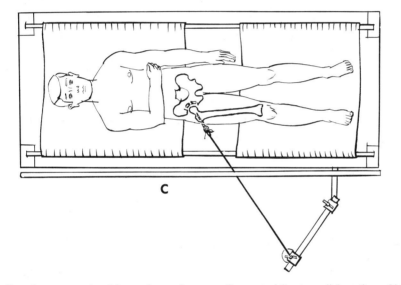

Fig. 42.   Traction on proximal femur by eyelet screw for central fracture dislocation of hip shown on a fracture bed with built-in Bradford frame to support the patient when the mattress is lowered for the bedpan.

Equipment

        1 long eyelet traction screw (inserted operatively)
        1 yd. of traction cord
        1 weight carrier and 15 pounds of weights
        1 base clamp assembly which can be attached to the undercarriage of the bed
        1 18-in. traction arm with end clamp
        1 9-in. traction arm with end clamp
        1 pulley with clamp assembly
        2 6-in. shock blocks

    Several skeletal traction alternatives are possible with a fracture dislocation of the hip. Traction may be exerted on the hip by a pin through the proximal tibia with balanced suspension as in Figure 31. The force is then exerted primarily in a longitudinal direction, depending somewhat upon the degree of abduction of the limb. This technique is advantageous if it is primarily the cephalic portion of the acetabulum that is crushed. Ninety-90° traction may be used as in Figure 40. This technique is useful if the injury is primarily a posterior fracture dislocation. Finally, traction may be exerted in a lateral direction by obtaining purchase on the proximal femur, preferably by a large eyelet screw inserted by operative technique similar to that used in nailing a fracture of the femoral neck. Purchase may also be obtained on the proximal femur by driving a Kirschner wire or Steinmann pin in an anteroposterior direction through the greater trochanter and out the lateral portion of the buttock, an undesirable system because of the large amount of soft tissues transversed.

All of these techniques are based on the hope that as the femoral head is repositioned, the acetabular fragments will follow it into their proper position under the influence of the stretched joint capsule and ligamentum teres and the relatively negative pressure created by extraction of the femoral head. If the acetabulum does not reconstitute itself, one may be able to replace and transfix the fragments surgically, particularly if they are few and large. Open surgery, however, cannot be performed without unjustifiable risk of infection if the patient has recently been treated with a percutaneous device in the proximal femur. For this reason, if it is anticipated that open reduction of the fractured acetabulum might be necessary, one of the alternate types of traction should be used regardless of which portion of the socket is shattered.

Unnecessary movement of the pelvis in patients who have recently sustained major fractures of any part of this structure is obviously undesirable. Partial sitting or turning of the patient is, of course, prohibited, and a fracture bed should be used to facilitate change of bed linen and use of the bedpan. The bed should be tilted to provide adequate countertraction and, in the cases of lateral traction, a bed side should be used.

References

DeWitt, R. F.: A method of treatment used in fracture of the acetabulum. J. Bone & Joint Surg., *24*:690, 1942.
Hamilton, F. G. and Cahoy, H. E.: The reduction of central fracture dislocations of the hip. Bull. Huron Road Hosp., *7*:4, 1961.

Through the Proximal Ulna for Fracture of the Humerus

Side arm

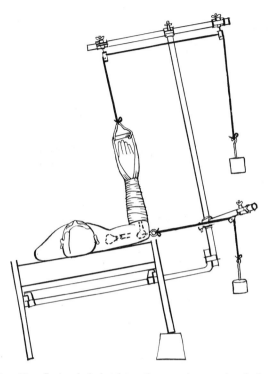

Fig. 43.   Lateral skeletal traction on the proximal ulna.

Equipment

1 Kirschner wire insertion tray or small eyelet traction screw (inserted operatively)
1 strip of commercial sponge traction tape or 1 long strip of moleskin or 3 long strips of 2-in. adhesive tape
1 3-in. elastic bandage
1 wire spreader with hand grip (Fig. 20)
2 yd. of traction cord
2 weight carriers and 15 pounds of weights
1 base clamp assembly which can be fastened to the undercarriage of the bed
1 36-in. traction arm with end clamp
1 27-in. traction arm with end clamp
1 9-in. traction arm with end clamp
3 pulleys with clamp assemblies
2 6-in. shock blocks

Occasionally it is desirable to treat a fracture of the humerus by skeletal traction. This situation prevails when it is anticipated that Dunlop's traction will prove inadequate for the treatment of a supracondylar fracture in a child. It also prevails in older children and adults with fractures of any part of the shaft of the humerus, if their general condition precludes either surgery or the use of an extensive cast or dressing. This situation frequently exists in patients with severe chest or abdominal injuries or with multiple fractures.

On the other hand, skeletal traction in these cases presents certain difficulties. Malalignment is sometimes difficult to correct, good alignment is difficult to maintain,

and motion at the fracture is difficult to prevent. For these reasons good patient cooperation must be obtained. He must remain flat on his back and as quiet as possible. Absolutely no sitting up can be tolerated unless the base clamp assembly can be attached
initially to the upper portion of the bedsprings rather than the main framework of the
bed. If the design of the bedsprings permits this modification, the patient's back rest
may be cranked up to a 45° angle provided there is no apparent alteration in the
orientation of the patient's arm to his trunk. A final and important difficulty is that if
skeletal traction should prove unrewarding, the situation cannot be safely salvaged by
surgical intervention owing to the proximity of the pin tract to the operative field.

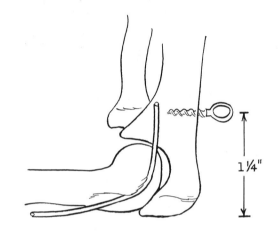

Fig. 44.   Preferred site for insertion of traction eyelet screw into the proximal ulna.

An eyelet screw, it seems, is the best means of obtaining traction on the proximal
ulna. To insert it securely it should be twisted into a small hole drilled in the cortex
opposite the coronoid process, where the greatest depth of bone is available. A small
incision is necessary for this procedure.

A Kirschner wire, driven transversely across the olecranon, is commonly used in
preference to a traction screw. However, it is difficult to insert without endangering
the ulnar nerve, sliding off the bone into a subperiosteal position, or transfixing part
of the joint capsule, with resultant elbow stiffness. The safest place for insertion is a
point on the bone halfway across the narrowest part of the ulna, where the olecranon
joins the body of the ulna. Driving the wire from medial to lateral aspects helps in
avoiding the ulnar nerve. One should resist the impulse to insert the wire across the
large prominence of the olecranon. So much of the palpable bulk of this structure is
the tendinous insertion of the triceps muscle that a traction wire in this region is likely
to lie in soft tissue rather than bone, a situation which, if unrecognized, can have
unpleasant consequences.

After the forearm is suspended by skin traction with the elbow flexed 90°, the limb
may be oriented in space by appropriate movement of crossbars and pulleys to align
the bone fragments in rotation as well as abduction and flexion (elevation). Occasionally it is necessary to align the fragments with their long axes vertically and with the
forearm suspended horizontally over the face. In this case the arrangement should be
switched to that illustrated in Figure 45.

When the traction is lateral rather than vertical, countertraction is best obtained by elevating the traction side of the bed on low shock blocks. In the author's experience an upper extremity Thomas traction splint incorporated in this arrangement offers no advantages and is usually quite troublesome.

Overhead

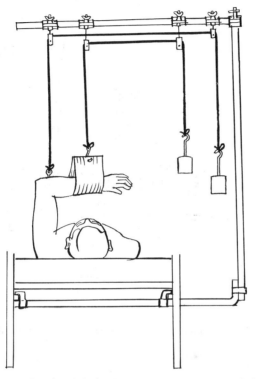

Fig. 45.   Overhead skeletal traction on the proximal ulna.

Equipment

    1 Kirschner wire insertion tray or small eyelet traction screw (inserted operatively)
    1 stockinette covered felt sling 10 by 14 inches (Fig. 15)
    4 yd. of traction cord
    2 weight carriers and 15 pounds of weights
    1 base clamp assembly which can be fastened to the undercarriage of the bed
    2 36-in. traction arms with end clamps
    4 pulleys with clamp assemblies

This arrangement may be preferred to the side arm counterpart described previously, particularly when the proximal fragment of the humerus is more adducted and flexed (elevated). No provision for countertraction is needed because of the vertical orientation of the traction force. Details of Kirschner wire or eyelet screw insertion are described in the preceding section. If counterweighted properly, the forearm sling facilitates some elbow flexion a..d extension with negligible disturbance of the fracture. Details of nursing care also are described in the preceding section.

Reference

McLaughlin, H. L.: Trauma. Philadelphia, W. B. Saunders Company, 1959.

Through Proximal Ulna and Through Distal Forearm or Hand for Combined Fractures of Humerus, Radius and Ulna

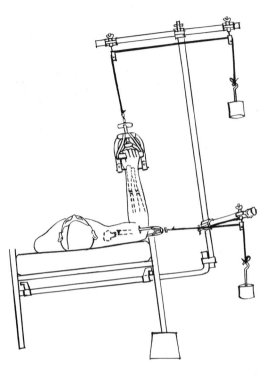

Fig. 46.   Skeletal traction on both proximal ulna and distal forearm.

Equipment

       1 Kirschner wire insertion tray and small eyelet traction screw (inserted operatively)
       1 6-in. section of broom stick or a bundle of 4 tongue blades for use as a hand grip
       3 yd. of traction cord
       2 weight carriers and 15 pounds of weights
       1 base clamp assembly which can be fastened to the undercarriage of the bed
       1 36-in. traction arm with end clamp
       1 27-in. traction arm with end clamp
       1 9-in. traction arm with end clamp
       3 pulleys with clamp assemblies
       2 6-in. shock blocks

When a fractured humerus is associated with a fractured forearm and for some compelling reason treatment by traction of the forearm as well as the humerus is necessary, skeletal traction is required. For this purpose the Kirschner wire is driven through the distal metaphyses of the radius and ulna or through various metacarpals.

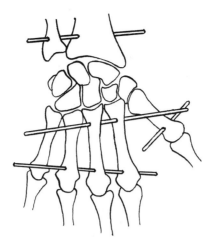

Fig. 47. Alternate locations for insertion of a traction wire through the distal radius and ulna or the metacarpals.

By careful insertion, direct injury to tendons can be avoided. However, in each case some degree of joint stiffness will prevail due to secondary inflammation of nearby tendons or other sliding structures. Therefore, whenever possible, some alternative such as open reduction and internal fixation should be sought.

Details of Kirschner wire insertion through the proximal ulna are described on page 50.

Cervical Traction by Skull Tongs

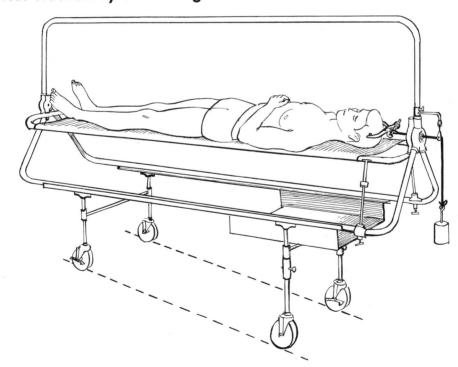

Fig. 48. Skull tongs used with a turning frame.

Equipment

        1 skull tong insertion tray
        1 yd. of traction cord
        1 weight carrier and 10–35 pounds of weights
        1 turning frame

In the presence of an unstable fracture or dislocation of the cervical spine, immediate immobilization of the neck is mandatory. The best method yet developed entails the use of some device that will secure skeletal traction on the skull. As mentioned previously, a head halter can substitute for calipers only temporarily because of the low tolerance of the underlying skin to pressure.

The various types of skull traction appliances in common use each have their own special features and adherents. The Vinke, Blackburn, and Barton devices are fixed into the parietal bones near the widest transverse diameter of the skull approximately 1 in. above the upper tip of the pinna of the ear. Vinke and Blackburn devices feature a flange on each of the tips of the points, designed to project between the inner and outer tables of the skull and thus prevent disengagement. In the author's experience, Vinke tongs are least likely to disengage but are technically more difficult to insert properly. Their application requires considerable time, a scrubbed-in assistant, and careful attention to the instructions shipped with the device. Since Barton and Crutchfield tongs lack flanges for engagement within the diploë, they must be tightened carefully for a few days after application to secure optimum seating of the points in the drill holes. It should be recognized that these tongs can be tightened too enthusiastically, leading to penetration of the inner table and hence occasionally to cerebral complications. Since Crutchfield tongs remain the most widely used, their insertion is described in detail in ensuing paragraphs. Except as already noted, the same principles of application may be applied to other devices.

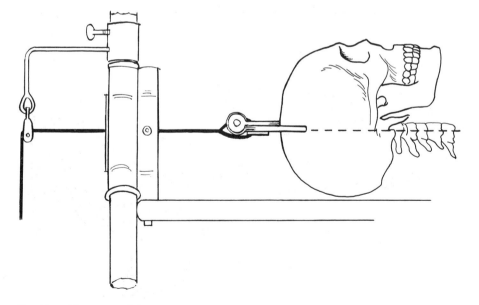

Fig. 49. Alignment of the tongs in the long axis of the cervical spine as indicated by the mastoid processes.

When necessary, an ordinary hospital bed may be used for tong traction. However, a turning frame such as the Stryker or Foster is much to be preferred as it permits turning the patient over and facilitates all other aspects of nursing care. If turning the patient is to be permitted, there is only one practical position for tongs and that position lies in the axis of the cervical spine as determined by the mastoid processes. When, for special fractures or dislocations, one wishes to apply traction with the neck flexed or extended, positions for the tongs slightly posterior or anterior, respectively, should be used. These modifications, however, render turning the patient difficult or impossible without reversing the bend of the neck, thereby neutralizing the effect desired.

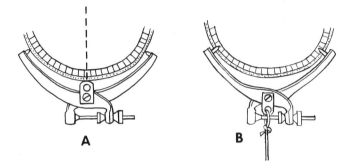

Fig. 50.   Localization of tong points by placing the traction cord attachment against the scalp in the mid-saggital plane.

The exact position for inserting the 2 points of the Crutchfield tongs is determined by rotating the metal loop for the traction cord 180° from its proper position for traction. The span of the tongs is then adjusted until the 2 points touch the scalp in line with the axis of the cervical spine at the same time the metal loop touches the scalp in the mid-saggital plane.

The Crutchfield tong insertion kit should include the following:

Prep. solution cups
Prep. sponge clamps
Sponges
Draping towels
Hypodermic needle and syringe
Scalpel blade and handle
Two small self-retaining retractors
Small periosteal elevator
Several small hemostats
Crutchfield drill tip with guard
Hand drill or brace
Crutchfield tongs
Several sutures with needles

This procedure is, of course, performed after the scalp has been shaved, cleaned and draped. Where each of the 2 tong points touches the scalp, the skin is infiltrated with a local anesthetic. A small cut is made down to bone, the incision is spread, the galea is cleaned off a small area of bone, and a hole is drilled through the outer table by use of a special drill tip with a guard to prevent penetration of the inner table. After the metal loop is rotated back to the traction position, the tong points are placed deep

in the holes and the locking nuts are tightened. If the incisions in the scalp are sufficiently large or bleeding, a stitch or two may be needed.

It is vital that the head end of the frame be elevated adequately to prevent the
patient from sliding up in bed and thereby neutralizing the traction. For this purpose
shock blocks are unnecessary, since the legs of these frames may be lengthened and
locked in place with special pins. During and after application of the tongs, the head,
of course, must not be moved unnecessarily lest neurologic injury occur.

References

Barton, L. G.: The reduction of fracture dislocation of the cervical vertebrae by skeletal traction.
    Surg. Gynec. & Obst., *67*:94, 1938.
Crutchfield, W. G.: Skeletal traction in the treatment of injuries to the cervical spine. J.A.M.A.,
    155:29, 1954.
Norton, W. L.: Fractures and dislocations of the cervical spine. J. Bone & Joint Surg., *44A*:115,
    1962.
Evans, D. K.: Reduction of cervical dislocations. J. Bone & Joint Surg., *43B*:552, 1961.
Vinke, T. H.: A skull-traction apparatus. J. Bone & Joint Surg., *30A*:522, 1948.

INDEX